Things Not To Say To Someone Who Has Cancer –

A Beginners Guide, Edition #1

© *Jo Hilder 2012*

Copyright Notice

Acknowledgements

To the many friends I've made along this journey because of cancer, some of whom are no longer here - "thank you". Knowing you changed me.

For the generous and amazing folks who allowed me to share their stories – thank you also. Names and some details have been changed to protect their privacy.

For Carol and Karl, and Tania, Tom and Vera.

To my wonderful cancer support group, who allowed me to plumb their depths and who supported me in my crazy dream to write a book about us and all we knew to be true: Margaret and Anne, Lynda, Mitch and Terri, Irena, Sandy, Avis, Ross, Gary, Peter, Janet, Paul, Karen, and Bill and Ann. We did something very special in the world, you know.

For Vanessa. ☺ You deserve a thank you all of your own.

For my friends and supporters at the Cancer Council NSW who encouraged, skilled and equipped me for this work, and for life, especially Patty, Anita, Kelly, Lorna, Annie, Carolyn and Meagan, and the team of co-facilitators at Living Well After Cancer. Words cannot express how grateful I am to all of you for the opportunities you've given me to help others with my story. Thank you for everything.

Thank you to Abigail Westbrook from **A Source Of Joy Graphic Design** for recreating the cover concept. Thank you also to Sallie Ann and Paul Macklin for ongoing support, inspiration and encouragement, and to Michelle Falzon for not allowing me to give up.

And to Ben, Beau, Levi, Daisy and Gabriel - For He knows the plans He has for us – plans to prosper us and not to harm us, plans to give us a hope and a future. - Jeremiah 29:11.

Table of Contents

Prologue

One day in July 2003 I woke up, got myself dressed, left home for work and didn't go home again at the end of the day. Instead, I went to hospital and stayed there. After several months of feeling unwell and being dismissed by my doctor as a hysterical, overworked middle-aged female, on this particular day I found out exactly what was wrong with me.

I had cancer.

In fact, I had a very big cancer. The tumour in my chest was the size of a saucer by the time it was found. My husband Ben took me to the emergency room at our local hospital where an x-ray revealed the huge mass behind my sternum. I was rushed to a bigger hospital in the next town, then flown to an even bigger hospital in the city where stage 3B Non-Hodgkin's Lymphoma was diagnosed. I started treatment immediately - three months of chemotherapy and two of radiotherapy - much of which I was obliged to have in a city four hundred kilometres away from my family and friends.

Besides those five months of treatment, several other things started the day I was diagnosed with cancer. A military-like operation, initiated by our church friends, designed to ensure Ben and our four children didn't starve while I was in hospital was one. With me away having cancer treatment for an undetermined period of time, the amazing and beautiful folks from our congregation and community rallied around my family with meals, housework and all kinds of wonderful messages of love and support. I'll always be very grateful for the help we received in those first difficult months.

Another thing that started when I found out I had cancer was an avalanche of messages and good wishes. Friends, relatives and people I hardly knew phoned and wrote, and sometimes even dropped by the hospital or our home to offer their support. It seemed everybody had something helpful they wanted to say. This was when it started to become interesting. Some of the things people wrote and said to me were wonderful and very encouraging. Some, however, were - well - not so much. I discovered there are specific things people like to say to a person who has cancer. I began to think there was a list posted somewhere, because different people were saying exactly the same phrases to me on a very regular basis.

"You know, I think God is trying to teach you something through this."

"There's a reason for everything that happens, you know."

"Good girl – you need to stay positive!"

"You'll be a better person when this is all over."

"If you *believe* and have enough faith, you'll be healed."

At first I just said 'thank you" or "I know", but then I began to think more deeply about these remarks. I realized I'd said exactly the same things to people before, but now I had time to think about them, I realized they didn't make much sense. Was God really trying to teach me something by giving me cancer? Was I definitely going to be stronger, or a better person afterwards? Did I really believe if I just prayed and had enough faith, the cancer would go away? Did anyone really believe any of the things they were saying?

I talked to other people who had cancer. Yes, since they were sick, they'd heard the same things too. And just like me before they'd had cancer they'd never given the things much thought. But since their diagnoses, some of the things people said to them about cancer had become an issue too, and even caused problems in their relationships. Why? Because once those particular things were said, nobody talked about how they really felt, or said what they really thought. In fact, the things people usually said to someone with cancer seemed to be like a very good way to quickly change the subject. Someone needed to explain how people with cancer did not want to hear the same old things any more, because sometimes we did not want to change the subject. Besides, some of the things being said were not true, and didn't help as much as people seemed to hope.

After noticing the similarities between my experience and that of others, I started writing about the things I thought we probably ought not say to someone who has cancer. At first, I wanted merely to bring the issue to people's attention and raise awareness. I wanted to explain how I thought the things we'd been saying to each other were redundant and not very helpful. Then I wrote a blog post about Things Not To Say To Someone Who Has Cancer. At the time I was still angry and frustrated, and pretty soon some other angry and frustrated people responded to what I'd written. They shared with me some of the things people said to them when they had cancer, and expressed how annoyed they were about them. In amongst all this griping and comparing of notes, every now and then someone would be brave enough to write and ask, "So, now I know what *not* to say - what **do I say** to someone who has cancer?" For a while, I didn't listen - I was busy airing all my grievances about the Things Not To Say. But after a while I realized it wasn't really good enough to just tell people what they shouldn't say. The essential problem wasn't being solved. *I'd raised awareness of the Things Not To Say To Someone Who Has Cancer, but I hadn't given people anything to say instead.* People weren't going to stop saying those old things to the person they loved who had cancer even if those things weren't very helpful, because they cared way too much to say nothing at all, and they didn't know what else to say. If I really wanted to help (and when I thought about it, I really did want to help) I needed to stop writing about Things Not To Say, and start working on a new message about things we could say to someone who has cancer instead.

I've spent many years since my own cancer went into remission in

2004 talking and listening to people who have cancer and running programs and support groups for people at various stages of their cancer journey. You can't do this work without coming to the conclusion people really are quite amazing - resilient and vulnerable, robust and sensitive, selfish and generous, all at the same time. When something like cancer comes along, it can bring out the very best and the very worst in us, just as the disease itself can have both terrible and transformative effects on those impacted by it. I've also learned when we don't know what else to do we will always just do the best we can, and sometimes that's exactly what's required in the situation. However, when we know *exactly* what to do, it's even better. It was never going to be enough for me to simply tell people what not to say and just hope they would be able to do better. I needed to finish my message.

Besides, there are other things I experienced when I had cancer I wanted to talk about. The impact of cancer on my life was far greater than just the physical. My diagnosis of advanced lymphoma and six subsequent months of aggressive treatment changed my life even though the treatment was successful in curing me. Post-treatment, I found my priorities changed. My goals and dreams were re-examined, reorganized and reinvented. My relationships were tried and tested, and some didn't weather the storm. My marriage broke down as I became wracked with anxieties and my husband slid into alcoholism. A couple of my closest friendships deteriorated for reasons I didn't fully understand. Everyone tried their hardest, but sometimes we were simply unable to make the best of ourselves available when someone else needed it the most. It was only much later I was able to process exactly what happened. It seems cancer didn't always make us all into better people, and when it was around not everything we did for one another was particularly heroic or praiseworthy.

Of all those relational problems arising from having cancer, more effective communication was probably the best answer to the worst of them. When my husband slumped into a deep depression brought on by the shock of my diagnosis and my two-month absence in treatment, he needed someone trustworthy he could talk to about his feelings of helplessness and despair. When one of my best friends accused me of being a neglectful mother right in the middle of my chemotherapy, we both needed a better understanding of one another's priorities. When at the end of my treatment I became filled with anxiety and unable to make the simplest of decisions, I needed a tribe of supporters who understood my new language and way of looking at the world. By the time it became clear the cancer wasn't coming back, I realized it wasn't the physical disease that had the greatest impact on my life. The changes to my relationships and my emotional and mental health post-treatment turned out to be far more significant and enduring issues than the actual cancer ever was.

With support, Ben and I were able to recover our marriage, and we've learned a lot about each other and ourselves from that time.

The fragility and complex nature of relationships means that when something like cancer comes along they can be stretched and tested, and sometimes even broken. At the same time, their robustness, prolificacy and capacity to evolve means that those relationships are potential solutions to many of our problems as well. In other words, while relationships can pose some baffling questions they can also turn out to be the answers to our problems, never more so than when we are buffeted with trials such as cancer.

When it comes to this guidebook, Things Not To Say To Someone Who Has Cancer was never just a snarky attempt to show how annoying some people can be when others are sick, or leave the pressing question about what they might say instead hanging in the air. My hope is we can find some new ways of thinking and talking about cancer, and in particular, new ways of talking to people who have it. This book is not merely a criticism, or an attack on people who want to help the person they care about who has cancer. It asks, "Considering the scope of problems cancer brings into our lives, can we find ways to communicate which mean our relationship is not one of them?" This to me is just as important as finding a physical cure for cancer.

In whatever situation you find yourself – a friend of a person with cancer, family member, neighbour, acquaintance, partner, parent, husband, wife or even carer - I want you to know this book is not picking on you. We've all said the Things Not To Say, and none of us meant to offend or upset anyone when we did. It's perfectly understandable reticence and fear can prevent us moving past those first awkward conversations. This book is my attempt to bring us all together on common ground so we can do whatever work cancer may require of us, be it physical, emotional, social or relational.

So here I stand in front of my eager group of learners, my whiteboard and a brand new red marker ready in my hand. *Welcome everyone* I say, and then draw a huge red circle on my board around the words *Things Not To Say To Someone Who Has Cancer*. I watch as you squirm uncomfortably in your chairs, while some blush self-consciously and others cross your arms and grow a little defensive. And it's at this point I say *well, I'm not locking the door, so you can leave anytime if you feel this is way too much, or maybe even too hard*. But you know what? I don't think you'll leave, because I believe in you, and because I know you care enough to stay. If we can push past these initial feelings of being confronted and challenged by the Things Not To Say, the work we do in facilitating better conversations will be preemptive to a deeper understanding of each other, which is what we all really need when one of us has cancer. So let me say thank you so much, and congratulations for signing on. I just know it will be worth it.

1

The "C" Word.
Common cancer clichés and why they don't help.

Cancer - it's one of the things in life we are most afraid will happen either to us, or to the ones we love. Cancer is also one of the final frontiers of medicine, which despite all our best efforts we've still failed to fully control or prevent. In 2003 when I was diagnosed, statistics stated that one in three people in the general population of the USA, Australia and the UK would be diagnosed in their lifetime. Now, just nine years later, in spite of millions of dollars spent on research into causes and prevention programs, it's now reported the incidence is more like one in two[*]. That's half your family. That's every second person you know. That's fifty percent of people in your workplace, church and neighborhood. And because every person diagnosed with cancer impacts the others around them in some way, what these statistics really mean is cancer affects every person in our community, in one way or another. Every. Single. Person.

Cancer Facts and Cancer Myths

But even though more of us are being diagnosed, more people are also surviving cancer. The Australian Cancer Institute[†] reports a

---

[*] http://www.cancer.org.au/Newsmedia/factsfigures.htm

drastic improvement in five-year survival[‡] rates over the last thirty years. In the 1980's, around half of people diagnosed with cancer survived. Now, two thirds of those diagnosed with cancer recover, and this is set to improve even further with rapid advancements in treatment, prevention and screening programs. Despite all this, a pall of terror and apprehension still surrounds cancer, exacerbated by the way we talk about it, and also the way we talk to and about the people who have it.

Brave. Victim. Fight. Battle. Hero.

Cancer, according to this particular set of nouns and verbs, is a violent, unseen and malevolent enemy, a living entity we engage against in a kind of war. Listening to this particular metaphor, we might expect having cancer is like being hunted, attacked or assaulted. Cancer is depicted as something that wounds, scars and disfigures, eating away flesh and bone before draining away all that is wonderful about us into nothingness. The way we talk about cancer, it's no wonder many people still feel a cancer diagnosis is overwhelming, and tantamount to being served with a death sentence.

I saw it on TV, so it must be true.

[†] http://www.cancerinstitute.org.au/news/i/more-people-surviving-cancer-in-nsw

[‡] The study extends only across the initial years following remission of disease.

Another reason we're so afraid of cancer is because of some very commonly held beliefs about what happens to people when they have it. However, cancer and treatment in real life is rarely the way it's depicted or talked about in movies or on television. For the most part, having cancer is not very interesting or exciting, and is far less heroic than you may have been led to believe. There are also dozens of false assumptions about what happens to you when you have cancer - losing your hair is one. Many people believe alopecia (loss of hair) is a side effect of the actual disease, which it isn't. It is a possible side effect of chemotherapy. But people having chemotherapy don't always lose their hair. Also, unlike what we see on TV, not everyone who has cancer has terrible pain all the time, is pale and emaciated, feels especially brave, and not everyone dies from it. Many people live long, productive lives after cancer, and a lot of people live with cancer and hardly anybody knows they have it. I hold the media responsible for perpetuating most of the cancer myths and broad generalizations we've come to accept as true. We've been largely brainwashed into thinking there is just one way to have cancer, but this isn't based on reality for most people. Everyone's cancer experience is different, and sometimes the hardest thing about having it is realising it's nothing like you thought it would be. I hope this book will go some way towards dispelling many of these cancer myths and help us all understand it, and those who are going through it, a little bit better.

I just want to help.

If you're reading this book it's probably because someone you know and love has been diagnosed with cancer and you want to help the best way you can. Just as importantly, you don't want to make things any worse than they already are. Now, before most of us ever have a chance to do anything practical or useful for our friend or loved one, we'll have a chance to *say something*. This is probably why you've chosen to read this book in the first place. Knowing what to do can be so much easier – after all, anyone can make a casserole or send flowers. But knowing what to say? That's a whole other matter. We know the power words have to make us feel good or bad, and nobody wants to make a person with cancer feel worse than they already do. So just as much as we need to know what not to say, we definitely need to know what to say instead.

I believe most people suspect the usual things we say to someone who has cancer are somehow *not quite right*. If we were all totally okay with them, we would never question them. But we do question them, and rightly so. Many are based on those cancer myths we've been programmed to believe, and not on the truth about having cancer or treatment and the way it affects our lives.

The standard list of things to say to someone who has cancer.

A cancer diagnosis elicits a range of verbal responses. When you have cancer, different versions of the same things are said to you so often it can almost seem like people are reading them from a list somewhere.

"These things are sent to try us."

"You're a fighter."

"What doesn't kill us makes us stronger."

"I think the Universe is trying to tell you something."

"Oh, my cousin had that, and they died."

"If anyone can beat this, you can."

This standard list of responses to cancer isn't written on a wall or in a book - it's in our heads. It's a fixed set of things to say to someone who has cancer we all seem to have, a list we've never really given much thought to. We may not even realize we have this list until we find ourselves in the situation calling for it. Having the list in and of itself is not a bad thing. We all have lists of things to say for different situations. How do these lists get there? We're making them all the time, starting when we're very young. Situational list-making is a social problem solving technique, a part of developing interpersonal and coping skills. In fact, it could be said acquiring various sets of responses for different situations is good mental health. There's nothing intrinsically wrong with having lists of things to say - in fact, the absence of appropriate responses might be considered far more of a problem. It is possible however to have too many things to say, and it's also possible to have a flawed list. Good responses to situations and problems foster deeper understanding between the people involved, and are both sensitive and logical. This is why most of the things to say on the standard cancer list don't help as much as we may think. Even though they are well intentioned and usually very kindly said, the standard responses are not particularly tactful, nor are they particularly logical.

They are what we might call *cancer clichés*.

"Everybody has to die of something."

Cancer clichés undoubtedly began as someone's genuine attempt to be helpful and encouraging, however most of them are largely untrue, erroneous and some are also in very poor taste. Now, before you become extremely offended and maybe even throw this book across the room, please know this:

If you've used a cancer cliché, the person you said it to probably understands it's because you really, really care and needed to say something to make things better.

For their part, most people with cancer truly understand when friends or family use a cancer cliché it isn't because of thoughtlessness. On behalf of people with cancer I'd just like to say *thank you for caring so much you said anything at all.*

What's wrong with cancer clichés?

Clichés are a natural and common part of language, a way of reducing the confusing and troubling things we face in life down to something more manageable. Sometimes, the use of a cliché is very effective for making something scary like cancer seem safe and innocuous.

"Cancer is a word, not a sentence."

Clichés are a language-based containment method, used because a cancer diagnosis can provoke some confronting questions. *How could something like this happen? What's going to happen next? Will this get worse before it gets better? Is this person going to die?* Using a cancer cliché conveniently and effectively heads off uncomfortable, unanswerable questions like these. But while clichés help us feel less threatened, they are also a kind of *final word*. They have the effect of bluntly shifting an uncomfortable conversation onto another topic: *so, now we've acknowledged that elephant in the room, let's talk about something else.* While clichés help us bring a conversation under control when we feel off our guard, they also convert open discussions into closed ones. They usually turn out to be the end of the discussion on the subject, yet clichés seldom answer the pressing question at hand.

Cancer clichés help us feel safe.

When we learn someone we love has cancer, we naturally feel both a pull towards and a push away from them. Our care and concern makes us want to draw closer, but at the same time, the anxiety caused by the cancer and its possible implications may also make us feel repelled. Clichés act as a kind of defense mechanism, protecting us against emotional threats, but what we may not be aware of is how the safe distance they create for us may feel to the other party. For the person who has cancer, the use of clichés can act as a kind of rebuttal, a signal this person intends to stay at a safe emotional distance away from us. This is not a very nice feeling.

So if clichés don't help, what is it a person with cancer needs from us right now?

Becoming comfortable with questions and not just answers.

Cancer is a question just screaming out for answers, but however frustrating it may be, unanswered questions are something we may need to become at ease with. Being close to a person with cancer is about learning to live with the fear cancer brings without tying off uncomfortable conversations with clichés. Clichés contain glimmers of truth, but in and of themselves *they are not truth.* Instead of feeling the need to resolve all these pressing dilemmas about life, death, illness and mortality, we need to allow the person having the cancer experience to find their own meaning and draw their own conclusions. The cancer is their experience, and while we are sharing it with them, they alone can decide how this looks and feels.

It's okay not to be positive all the time.

Many times, people use cliché's simply because they have a need to fill the air with what they think is upbeat, positive talk. Chatter of any kind means there is no room left for scary silences or unanswerable questions. However, when you're with someone who has cancer there is really no need to feel as though you have to talk all the time, or otherwise responsible to brighten things up every time you appear on the scene. It's okay for a person with cancer not to be positive sometimes, and they may be waiting for a chance not to have to appear brave or strong. Being expected to be a hero all the time is a huge responsibility.

Also, it's perfectly all right for you to not know what to say. You can just say, "I don't know what to say." You'll probably know exactly what to say once you hear what they have to say first. Listen for any cues that may prompt you to know what they would like to talk about, and listen as well for any needs you may be willing and able to meet. Being a person who listens is going to be far more useful than being someone who feels the need to be the bearer of eternal sunshine and happiness all the time.

Be unwilling to let cancer define anyone or anything.

When you have cancer, it can become the single most defining event in your life. Some people, especially clinicians and health professionals, even identify you personally by the cancer you have. It's also common for people to identify cancer survivors as a certain type of person - stronger and more "down-to-earth" somehow - but this isn't always so. Cancer doesn't always make people stronger, or even make them into better people. I'll discuss this in a later chapter, because other peoples expectations can be a very difficult part of going through cancer, especially if others feel you ought to be a more resilient and more highly-evolved person simply because you had a disease.

Be gracious.

As a person caring for someone with cancer, you'll naturally feel fragile emotionally at times, but try not to be too brittle. It's important to practice supporting each other as the confronting or frightening conversations unfold, allowing and facilitating the exploration of what may be huge, life-changing subjects. Don't keep records of minor offenses or infractions. These are exceptional circumstances, and it may take exceptional grace and compassion for you to get through them.

Be yourself, and be realistic.

You bring to this relationship and to this experience unique insights and perspectives all your own. Trust those things about yourself. Don't try and be all the things you think your loved one needs, or try to be something you're not. There will be a role for you in all of this, and while it may take a little time for you to settle into it, you'll work it out. Be who you are, and remember - you're stronger, wiser and smarter already than you probably realize.

Also, remember you're not anyone's savior. You're human, and you can only do so much. Don't overcommit yourself physically or emotionally from a sense of guilt or obligation, or because you're a "doing" type of person and you feel like you can't help yourself.

———

Think carefully about the level of commitment you're realistically able to give to this situation right now. You may need to make some very tough decisions, and we'll discuss this further in future chapters.

The best thing to say is probably not something to say.

Perhaps the very best thing you can offer your friend is to simply be yourself. Be a listener, an ally and a sounding board. Be kind, be gentle and be generous, and not just to your friend – when someone you love has cancer, you'll need to be all these things to yourself as well.

Come with me.

In the book that follows, I'd like to talk to you about saying and doing things for your loved one with cancer in ways that will make a positive difference. I know this is what you've come looking for. I also want to foster an atmosphere where some new kinds of cancer conversations can occur, both spoken and unspoken. I'd like to explore new ways of talking about cancer because I know no matter who, what or where we are, at some time cancer *will* come into our lives, and it would be great if cancer brought something other than the fear, terror, anxiety and misunderstanding it so frequently brought before. I believe cancer can be an opportunity for us to create and recreate better relationships, conversations and dialogues. I like to see cancer as an opportunity to find new ways of understanding each other, and of inventing new, creative avenues for giving and receiving love, kindness and compassion. What if, instead of sending us on a search for old ways of talking and thinking and being, cancer caused us to search our own feelings and beliefs, helping us answer those old fears with new hope and new appreciation for life? Whilst we strive to create a society without cancer in our generation, I believe in using as many resources to seek better and more creative ways to stop cancer from destroying us in a thousand terrible ways whilst ever it remains with us. Will you join me?

2

Getting Your Head Around Things To Say
To Someone Who Has Cancer.
The first conversation.

For many people, the first conversation after a cancer diagnosis is the most difficult part of the entire journey. Some of us will be well prepared for it, others not so much. There are definite ways we can ready ourselves mentally and emotionally, but no matter how ready we think we are, it can still be extremely daunting.

Several weeks ago, a woman came into the shop where I work looking for a gift for her friend. I could see she was close to tears, and it didn't take long before she revealed to me the reason. It seems the friend she was buying for was diagnosed with cancer several months before, but her terrified friend still hadn't been able to bring herself to visit. Her emotion spilled over as she shared with me her abject fear of saying or doing the wrong thing in her friends' presence. In her mind, her friend had become like a saintly entity she was fearful of offending with her fumbling and emotional gestures. Her apprehension was so strong she had managed to avoid any contact with the friend for quite some time, but her conscience finally motivated her to call and make a date. I helped her choose a small gift, encouraging her not to worry about it - I was sure her friend would just be extremely pleased to see her. She was filled with shame at having avoided visiting for so long, and felt as a result their friendship might be permanently affected. In succumbing to her overwhelming fear of losing this friend to cancer, she risked losing the friendship to neglect in the meantime.

It's difficult to judge this woman for her actions, as her fearful response to her friends' cancer diagnosis surely resonates with most of us. But whether you jump right in or hold back indefinitely, there simply has to be this very first conversation with your friend or family member after they've been diagnosed with cancer, and you can surely be forgiven for being nervous about it. The first time we speak with them will probably be when we feel the most pressure to say something to make them instantly feel better. This is when you'll be digging around back there in your mind, trying to find ways to pull this cancer thing into some kind of shape in your head and make it feel safe and small and less powerful.

Just a heads up - *this first contact after the diagnosis is when you're most likely to use a cancer cliché.*

Whether the cancer diagnosis has only just happened or it's been some time since, here are two common issues you're likely to confront.

"I just need to say something."

Last weekend, I was talking to my mother about writing this book, and she mentioned how a few days beforehand she had gone to a store she frequents and glimpsed a female employee who hadn't been there for a while. As my mother approached the counter where the employee was standing she noticed the woman was wearing a headscarf and had missing eyebrows. Realizing what had probably happened since they last chatted, my mother tentatively asked her "How are you?" The woman explained she had recently been diagnosed with breast cancer and was having chemotherapy, and in the week before had lost all her hair. "And after that," my mother explained to me, "I was stuck. I had no idea what to say next. I wanted to say how both my sister and my daughter had cancer and I knew how she felt, but that was just words. I don't know how she feels. I felt like in that moment, I really needed something else I could say."

Most people find themselves in this position when faced with a person with cancer. Cancer is like the virtual elephant in the room, inspiring both fear and apprehension and is almost impossible to ignore. We don't know if the person with the cancer is expecting us to acknowledge the topic up front, or if they will be offended because we deliberately don't mention it. My mothers question, "How are you?" can be a good opener, except for the fact the scripted response is "Good!" Commonly, we don't expect someone to respond to this particular enquiry with how they really feel, especially if it isn't good. The woman my mother was speaking to clearly understood her question to be a cue for her to explain her appearance, and took the opportunity to respond honestly.

However, stumped for something else to say, my mother simply left it there, which was probably the most appropriate response given the fact they are not close friends. In informal conversations like this one, the person who doesn't have cancer can feel they are supposed to make the person with cancer feel instantly comfortable. Please know there is not really anything you can say which will serve this purpose, because cancer is never going to be one of those things we feel really comfortable talking about, particularly at first. Sometimes the right thing to say is nothing at all. A genuine, shocked silence is at the very least perfectly honest.

"I need to provide some kind of answer to the problem."

Cancer is nothing if not a big, scary question. But you don't have the answer. The person with cancer doesn't have the answer. None of us have the answer. The answer is found in a test tube somewhere, or is perhaps still locked away inside some exotic seed in the Amazon. But whatever and wherever all those cures are for all the different kinds of cancer, the cliché's we throw around every time we hear the word uttered do absolutely nothing to help.

When confronted with a person who has cancer, it's normal to feel like you need to have something authoritative to say. We want to diminish cancer, reduce it down and make it into something we can make go away with just one glib sentence. But that's not going to happen. But while there are no simple answers for something as formidable as cancer, there are steps we can take to move us through it and out the other side.

———

Don't talk.

Rather than assuming what your loved one really needs from you is an answer for cancer, consider this. What if instead of talking, you simply listened? Instead of trying to think of answers, what if you placed your focus on hearing what – if anything – they have to say about cancer, or any other thing they may want to talk about?

What if instead of trying to provide closed answers, you asked open-ended questions? Instead of stating clichés designed to close cancer down, what about asking questions which have more than one kind of reply, and instead of leading the conversation, you allowed them to do so?

What are open questions?

The best way to facilitate a generous and interesting conversation is with open questions. Open questions are questions you don't already have the answers to.

"What's happening for you at the moment?"

"How are you feeling about what's going on right now?"

"Where is everything up to?"

"What's next for you?"

Conversely, questions you perhaps already know the answers to, or which can be answered with just a "yes" or a "no" are *closed questions*. Examples of closed questions might be –

31

"Are you scared?"

"Does it hurt?"

"Do you need chemotherapy?"

"Are you having surgery?"

There's only one way to answer these questions, and so there's only one way this conversation can go. From here on in, you'll be talking about cancer whether either of you wants to or not, because the questions up to this point lead directly into it. But what if one or both of you doesn't want to talk about cancer? Asking questions that can lead either to or off topic will open up the conversation and not close it down.

The examples of open questions I have given above are not cancer specific, and they give the person a chance to guide the conversation away from cancer if they want to. Any of these questions could just as easily end up being about what's happening with the kids at school, what their plans are for the weekend or what they did at work. Asking open questions has the added benefit of making you into a safe and interesting person to be with. If you move the focus away from cancer and don't allow it to become and stay the center of attention, your friend will know you *see them as a person* before you see them as someone with a disease.

An important point – particularly for a casual or first contact with a person who has cancer - you only need ask a couple of questions, not twenty. More than a few questions will feel like an interrogation. Your role is to help both of you relax, and provide just enough cues for a good conversation to start, if appropriate. Any curiosity you are feeling can be satisfied in various other ways perhaps at another more opportune time.

What do you do when you've exhausted a couple of open questions? If it's your very first meeting after the diagnosis, it may mean it's time for you to go. Again, listen to your friend, and watch for body language. Don't outstay your welcome. If this is a casual conversation, as it was for my mother and her acquaintance at the store, perhaps one open question is enough to convey sincere concern without letting that elephant in the room take over the conversation altogether.

Warning – asking open questions may be dangerous!

The whole purpose of asking open questions is to start a conversation with the person who has cancer – but you need to remember this may turn out to be a *conversation about cancer. Oh no!* I hear you say. *But I don't want to talk about cancer! I don't want to hear them talk about cancer either!* Perhaps very unfortunately for you, I'm working from the assumption that you won't mind engaging with someone who has cancer in a conversation about cancer. I could be completely wrong about that. The idea may absolutely terrify you.

If the idea of talking about cancer makes you anxious, perhaps this is a good time for you to have a think about exactly why that is. Does cancer bring up negative memories for you, perhaps recollections of a painful past experience with another person? Do you not know enough about cancer or the impacts of it to feel comfortable discussing it? Perhaps you have some preconceptions or assumptions and you're acting on those? Maybe you think this person will expect something of you that you feel ill-equipped to give them?

Before you make initial contact with the person who has cancer, you may need to do a little soul-searching to try and understand what your own feelings and beliefs may be concerning cancer. If you have a personal cancer experience of your own, or a person you cared for died from cancer, its understandable your emotions and memories may be triggered by this context. It doesn't mean something is wrong with you - it may simply mean that you need just as much comforting and compassion as your friend with the cancer does right now, and it may be something which needs your attention.

It may help you to remember positive relationships with other people are an essential part of healthy cancer treatment. While you can't do much about your loved ones physical sickness or their pain, you can certainly do something about the positive relationship side of things by doing your best to see they have one with you.

Prepare yourself.

Have a little talk with yourself about any preconceived thoughts and feelings you may have about cancer, and try to disconnect those from the person you're about to see. Be prepared to feel a little awkward at first. Something pretty big happened since last you saw each other, so regardless of how they may appear, things may not be entirely as they once were. If you haven't seen them for a while, be prepared to see your friend totally changed, or even apparently unchanged. Either way, you may be in for a surprise.

Be conscious of your facial expressions and the tone of your voice. You are not attending their funeral or about to deliver their eulogy. Also, if you were merely acquaintances beforehand, be mindful you have not suddenly become the best of friends. They may not appreciate overt physical contact or familiarity. A good tip is to remember to relate to them now as you would have related to them before this happened.

Don't expect too much from yourself, because this person may not be expecting as much from you as you think. By the time most people have their head around having cancer they realize most of their friends and family are feeling as helpless and anxious as they are. But while it's okay to feel upset and feel anxious and helpless, try not to bring those feelings with you and dump them on your friend like it's their job to make you feel better about the cancer. Also, you will not prove how much you care by escalating the level of your emotion in their presence. Sometimes the most generous gift you can bring a person with cancer is your own emotional stability. When you have cancer, you sometimes feel as though you have to be cheerful because you seem to make everyone else feel so terrible. Of course, there may be moments when you're together and emotions may run high. I'm not advocating being hard of heart, stoic to a fault or pretending you don't care. But don't throw your hands up and rail *"Why? Why? Why?"* You can be sure they don't have the answer, and it may be they are wondering why, why, why you came at all today, when clearly what you really needed was a half-hour of professional counseling and a nice cup of tea.

Let them do the talking, at least at first.

Make up your mind that you'll be letting your friend or family member do most of the talking until it's clear what the "ground rules" are. They may be happy for you to talk and just sit back and listen, but don't assume the empty spaces between you are there for you to fill up. Prepare yourself to sit in silence if required. Also, arrive in a relaxed, present state of mind. A cup of chamomile tea before you go is a good idea, but three cups of coffee? Not so much. Where it is within your power, set this up to be a meeting without complexity, pressure or stress, for your own sake and for your friends.

What's going to happen?

You'll be doing lots of listening. When you do talk, you'll be asking a couple of open questions so your friend can lead the conversation wherever they want it to go. In fact, if you have a job as a support person, it's to open up the conversations and keep them open. Your job isn't to talk about cancer in terms of what you know about it, what you think you know about it and what you think should be done, because it doesn't actually matter what you think or know about their having cancer. *What matters is what they think and know about it.*

Of course, you have your own questions. You want to know what's going to happen next, what treatment they'll be having and what their prognosis is. However, don't interrogate your friend with a barrage of questions about their treatment or the disease. They'll tell you what they want you to know. You can always read up in your own time. When I had cancer, Ben gave everyone close to us a brochure about Non-Hodgkin's Lymphoma so they knew exactly what kind of cancer I had. I recommend you snoop around your hospital oncology department or ask a cancer charity[§] for some information or literature to read. Beware of searching for information on the Internet. A great deal of the information available online about cancer and treatments is from unreliable

[§] The Cancer Council NSW provides a free Cancer Helpline on 13 11 20 (within Australia) providing information on cancer and treatment, peer support (patient to patient, telephone & online), support groups, referrals to free legal and financial planning services as well as information on Cancer Survivor programs. Qualified oncology nurses are available between the hours of 9am to 5pm. The Cancer Council NSW can also send out free information brochures on most kinds of cancer and the available treatments. Call the helpline on 13 11 20 (within Australia) for more information.

sources, may not be evidence based and is unverifiable for accuracy, clinical or otherwise.

Don't be the expert, the know-it-all or the fixer.

Let go of any expectations you may have of your friend with cancer. Don't go expecting you'll be required to rush in and "fix" everything. You may be in for a surprise.

Make up your mind you'll try not to fill the empty air with chat, instead looking for cues on what they want to talk about. They may not even want to talk about cancer. They may want to talk about something else completely. They may however want to tell you absolutely everything. They may not know how much you know already, and they might be looking for a signal from you to indicate what you do know. Tell them how much you already know, but don't tell them all of what you *think* you know. In other words, don't make yourself the cancer expert. If you use open questions, you're sure to have the conversation they feel most comfortable having.

Presents and gifts.

Now, concerning gifts. If you must take something with you on your first visit, here are a few suggestions –

- **Something green and living**. Plants and flowers are good, but check first, particularly if they're in hospital, as many

---

38

people having chemotherapy cannot tolerate flowers in the room and the hospital may not permit them.

- *Chocolate* is also good, or else their favorite candy or sweet. A bottle of wine, where appropriate, is fine. Even if they cannot eat the chocolate or drink the wine, they can share it with their visitors or family.
- *A book by a favorite author.* Do not however take a cancer curing diet book. Do not take a printed copy of that spam email about cancer. Do not take any props, visual aids or other random things alluding to miraculous cures or morbid causes of cancer, unless you have been very specifically asked for them.
- *An empty journal.* And a lovely pen to write with.
- *Something they want but can't get.* They may already have a clear idea of something they want but are having trouble getting their hands on. This may be something you can assist with.

As for ongoing practical support, gifts and presents in the post-diagnosis phase, I'll go deeper into this subject later in the book.

Note - do not use your first visit as an opportunity to evangelize, "witness" to your friend about a particular God, or try to convert them to a religion, diet, or spiritual practice.

This is not your big chance to witness or evangelize, convert them, sell them something, or air your spiritual theories about cancer, including whether or not cancer is the Universes way of trying to teach them something. Don't preach, and don't bring your Bible or other spiritual book with you to refer to while you talk. If you have a burning need to sermonize or philosophize about your friends' cancer, I suggest you start a blog or buy yourself a blank journal. And keep it to yourself. *Seriously*. Because I believe it's important, I'll go further into this subject later in the book.

Confirm it's convenient to visit, and when you arrive, keep it brief.

Decide beforehand you will not overstay your welcome. Call before to confirm the time, and check today is a good day to come by. Once you arrive, make it clear you haven't planned to stay all day. It's better to be invited to stay longer than asked to leave early. Go in pairs or in a group where appropriate, but don't ever take someone along with you for your own moral support the person you're visiting has never met before. They are not something interesting for you both to look at and then discuss later over lunch. If you need to take your children with you, please ask if it's okay before you turn up with them in tow. Most of this is common courtesy.

As you leave, ask if and when you might visit again. If you make a date, write it down, and tell them you'll call them to confirm.

In all the ways that really count, the person you love who now has cancer probably hasn't changed that much. They may be hoping you are the one bringing that fresh face of normality, and also hoping your relationship is one of the few things in life that hasn't been disrupted by cancer. And as scary as cancer is, as much as it's within your power you can do something about that. If you've decided to walk their cancer journey with them, do it by making up your mind your relationship will not be one of the things cancer changes…unless, of course, it's for the better.

It's all too much.

Sometimes we hold back emotionally or physically simply because we don't want to let the person down. We may feel our best may not be enough, or that we'll fail the one we love right when they need us most. Just this morning I missed a phone call from a friend whose husband was admitted recently to a hospital very close to our home. Listening to her quick voicemail message, I felt an immediate apprehension about phoning her back. Was she going to ask me if she could stay with us while her husband was in the hospital? Did she just want to catch up for a coffee while she was so close by? My mind was racing, thinking about whether I would be able to accommodate what she might be expecting. Soon afterwards, I felt guilty for being so reticent. Surely if I were a good friend I'd call her back without hesitation? A short time later, as I was thinking about writing this chapter, it occurred to me what I was feeling this morning is the same as many people feel before going to visit their loved one with cancer. We assume it's going to be too much for us to handle, and we fear we won't be able to cope with what we hear or see. We could however be overestimating others expectations of us - emotionally, logistically and relationally - or we may even be underestimating our own capacity to help. Our apprehension is normal and we needn't feel guilty. Sometimes it's a matter of having a little bit of faith in ourselves and in the quality of our friendship, and a little less faith in cancers power to bring chaos into our lives.

Grace, grace and more grace.

I'd like to end this chapter with a few home truths, and an act of grace. You need to know that when it comes to "being there" and saying the right things to a loved one who has cancer, you're probably not going to get it right all the time. You may mess it up occasionally, even if it's just in small ways. You may even mess it up in a big way, but you'd be pretty darn unlucky if you did. You may say the wrong thing – it may only be once, but chances are you'll do it. You may do something you think is a great idea which later turns out not to be, or perhaps not do something you later regret and wish you'd done. You'll say yes and wish you'd said no, and say no, wishing afterwards you'd said yes. You'll decide you can't handle this and then find out later you probably could. You'll think it's far worse than it turns out to be, and you'll also underestimate how significant it really is. The bottom line is – and this is what I really want you to remember - *you're only human.* There is no perfect or one right way to cope with having a loved one with cancer – you'll just have to make most of it up as you go along. You're bound to blow it sometimes. And that's okay.

Really, it's okay.

This I know: what I'm about to suggest, you can do right now, or much later if you want to, but sooner or later you'll just have to do it.

Forgive yourself.

You are not perfect. Pardon all your own flaws, your shortcomings and your mistakes. Trust your motives, and don't carry guilt or shame because perhaps you weren't able to shine as brightly as you hoped. You may just surprise yourself, if not this time, then maybe next time.

Things to remember -

- *It's perfectly normal to feel apprehension about your first meeting after the diagnosis. If you need to put it off until you feel more comfortable, do so, but don't wait to get together so long the friendship is placed under strain.*

- *When you do meet, your job is to listen and to ask open-ended questions.*

- *Inform yourself about their cancer by reading information in your own time from trustworthy sources.*

- *Call to confirm, take a thoughtful gift, and keep your first meeting brief unless invited to stay longer.*

- *Remember, if you inadvertently blow it or commit a faux pas, it isn't the end of the world. Apologize, forgive yourself, and move on.* ☺

3

Do-ers, Feelers and Thinkers
Three most common responses to the news someone has cancer.

About six months after I finished my cancer treatment and went into remission, I found out that Sharon, a regular customer to my shop and a fellow stitcher, was diagnosed with bowel cancer. Over a period of several months her belly had become more and more bloated, and, upon finding what they thought was a benign tumor on the ovary, her doctor scheduled her for surgery. But instead of removing an innocuous lump as they'd planned, they found they were dealing with a well-advanced malignancy - way too much cancer too be operable - the worst possible news.

Sharon's close friend Mandy came to see me the day she found out. Mandy was clearly in shock as she shared what they knew so far. Sharon was due to start chemotherapy later that week, a treatment not expected to cure her but perhaps prolong her life - a little. I tried to comfort Mandy, reassuring her Sharon was in the best possible hands: I knew the team looking after her personally - they were quality clinicians. I knew better than to offer Mandy any pat answers. It was awful, and there wasn't any way around it. But Mandy didn't want to stand around and wring her hands about how awful it was, any more than I wanted to placate her. She didn't want to talk about what this meant in the bigger scheme of things, or even if Sharon's treatment was likely to work. "Just tell me what I can *do*, Jo," she said. "Tell me what needs to be done, and I'll go do it." I suggested Mandy visit the social worker at Sharon's oncology ward and collect some information on the impacts of chemotherapy, both for herself and Sharon's other friends. We both knew it wasn't much, but it gave Mandy a kind of mission to send herself on. Mandy didn't want comforting, counseling or even a shoulder to cry on. What Mandy really wanted was *something to do*.

Just a few weeks ago, I went to have coffee with a few friends. I was catching up with one particular girlfriend for the first time in about ten years - we certainly hadn't seen each other since I'd been sick. Just as the others were starting to leave, Allie pulled me aside, whispering that she had something she needed to tell me. As we sat down around the corner of the table, Allie took my hands in hers and said solemnly "I feel I need to ask your forgiveness for something."

"Allie, we haven't seen each other in nearly a decade. What could you possibly have to be sorry to me about?"

"I am so sorry because when I found out you had cancer, I did nothing for you. I didn't write, I didn't call - nothing. I wanted to, I thought about it so many times, but every time I thought about you, all I could do was get upset and cry. It overwhelmed me. I got lost in all of that emotion, and it kind of paralyzed me. In the end, I just couldn't reach out, because my feelings about how awful it was were too much. I had to decide not to think about you at all or I'd just go around crying all the time." I thanked Allie for her honesty, and let her know there was nothing to be forgiven. In fact, I was grateful Allie hadn't reached out to me in her distress. I remembered how I'd often felt confused, and what I really needed in those times was a stable shoulder to lean on. But also, knowing how deeply my situation was touching other people was a kind of validation, both of the situation I was in and of the depth of their regard for me. *This really is as bad as I think it is, and they really do care about me.* My touching conversation with Allie reminded me that many times, a person close to someone diagnosed with cancer is overcome by their own *feelings and emotions.*

Wendy and I were friends for a long time by the time I found out I had cancer. We shared numerous homeschooling connections, church connections and writing connections. Wendy at that time lived in New Zealand and I lived in Australia, so we were only able to see each other in person maybe once a year. When Wendy received news about my having cancer, she knew just what to do. She sent an email to her contacts all over Australia, New Zealand and the world, telling them about me and asking them to pray. She asked several of our mutual friends to help put together a scrapbook of beautiful pictures and bible verses she planned to send to me in hospital. She contacted several of her friends in Sydney and asked if they would be available to visit me in hospital. In those first few weeks, with Wendy in another country and me without mobile phone credit or access to the Internet or email, she and I barely spoke to one another. But every now and then I would receive mail from someone I'd never met. "Wendy told us about you" the card would say, "and we're praying for you." When I was in hospital, I received phone calls from Wendy's friends – would I like a visitor? I need only say yes, and Wendy's friends would be there for me. Wendy's non-intrusive thoughtfulness was wonderful because it required I do nothing, say nothing, give nothing and be nothing else other than what I was. Wendy is a perfect example of someone who converted her deep and sincere *thoughts of care and concern* into practical assistance.

When I look back at the first few weeks of my diagnosis, I recognize the wide variation in the reactions of the people I knew. And why wouldn't they be different? Every person, every friend, relative and acquaintance is different in personality, beliefs and personal experiences. If two members of the same family can react to the same situation in varying ways, it shouldn't really surprise us that something as frightening as cancer can make people respond so differently.

Most people will react initially to the news that someone they know or love has been diagnosed with cancer with a sense of shock and disbelief. It's often unexpected news, and to added to that, it's also bad news. Whenever any of us is faced with unexpected and bad news, we usually act more from reflex than reason, perhaps even with a *fight or flight* response. Most people settle down after a short amount of time into a kind of coping mechanism, commonly in one of the three categories typified by Mandy, Allie and Wendy. You may find you identify with one of these three types of responses.

Do-ers. Doing people like Mandy are not satisfied to just wait around for news or wring their hands. They are deeply motivated to find something practical to do, and usually see obvious needs they can easily meet. Achieving these objectives helps alleviate their own anxiety about the situation, and if channeled appropriately, can meet some tangible needs of the person with cancer. Most people feel obliged to help in some way, but do-ers make it their goal to see real results from their actions, and may even commit to leading or facilitating a long-term practical plan of support. Do-ers need lists, tasks and identified needs they can strategize and plan around, and may need some firm direction, because if left to their own devices can become intrusive or misdirected. Because they are the ones with the confidence, energy and resources to get things done, if given the information they need, do-ers can make a person with cancer's life much, much easier.

If you are a doing type of person, try to remember to take your cues from the person you want to help or their direct circle of concern. Don't barge in uninvited or make assumptions. If you are not within their immediate circle of concern, take any ideas you may have to the ones closest to them and ask which if any you may facilitate. You may need to wait for direction if things are busy, or they don't seem to know what's going on. Make any offers non-intrusive and realistic, and be careful not to overcommit yourself. Also, be clear on what your expectations are for being thanked, because these kinds of reciprocations can sometimes become lost in translation. Giving time and energy to a complex situation like cancer can seem like a one-way street at times, and can call for some stamina and sacrifice. Pace yourself, and remember to look after your own. If possible, put a small team of helpers together, or become part of a team that already exists so you don't burn out. As a do-er, you are a wonderful asset to any situation, and your talent and energy may turn out to be a huge blessing in a time like this.

Feelers. While everyone will feel shock and distress at news of the cancer, deep-feeling people will be particularly heartbroken. They will ruminate over the situation and fully explore any implications of loss and change. Like Allie, the strength of their emotions may overwhelm them, and they may cry a lot, and may need to talk to someone outside of the situation about it. This is certainly more desirable than unburdening any anxiety and distress onto the person with the cancer. While there may be times when you will have a cry with the person who has the cancer, these particular circumstances dictate that one of you is the person who needs most of the support right now, and the other is the person who will be doing most of the supporting. A support person certainly needs to feel empathy, but if you find you're relying on your loved one with cancer to do most of the comforting, it may be time for you to seek a support person of your own.

Feelers can be the most awesome people to have around. When other people may be bothering you with endless questions and pep talks, a well-centred feeling person is someone you can just be yourself with. When you're ready to talk about how it really feels to be a person with cancer, they'll be the ones who want to know about it. The strength of their emotional investment in your experience is also incredibly validating. While others are telling us to think positive and promising us everything is going to be okay, feelers help remind us there is a real, living person inside this cancerous body who *feels something,* and it isn't always positive or brave. By affirming our feelings and emotions, feelers help us remember we are more than just a cancer patient when we're being poked, prodded and talked about as if cancer is the most interesting thing about us.

Unfortunately feelers don't always think themselves capable of the kind of compassionate support they'd like to offer. Like Allie, deep feelers often avoid contact with the person involved altogether because they feel inadequate, or fear they will not be able to control their own emotions. Deep feelers can go to great lengths to avoid any meetings simply because they can't deal with the power of their own sadness and grief. As a result they may appear aloof or uncaring when in fact the opposite is true. This can be particularly difficult if the deep-feeling person doing the avoiding is a very close family member or friend of the person with cancer. Many misunderstandings have occurred between a person with cancer and someone they love dearly, simply because one of them seemed to pull away at a time when they other expected they would draw close. Having an insight into your predisposition to powerful or incapacitating emotions may help you explain to your loved one with cancer what you're feeling, and why you cannot be there for them right at this moment. Communication is the key to avoiding most misunderstandings in times like these.

Thinkers. For most of us being confronted with something like cancer can seem like pressing the pause button. Our thought processes freeze - everything comes to a grinding halt. Some things are different than they were before, and some are the same, but until we work out which is which we don't really know how to move forward. Thinkers like Wendy see things differently. Wendy viewed my having cancer as a series of opportunities, a bunch of loose ends all with logical partners somewhere - she just had to find them and join them up. Thinkers have a kind of mental filing cabinet in their mind all stocked up with ideas and strategies and contact details, and when something in life moves out of place somewhere, they open that cabinet and get busy pulling files and making calls.

Thinkers like Wendy are great at strategizing, but they don't necessarily end up carrying out all their own plans. They usually have a mental note up there on exactly who is good at what, and can activate those contacts at a moments notice. If you give them a problem, they'll go and work out a solution to it, recruiting and motivating volunteers as they go. On learning I had cancer, Wendy concluded my most pressing problem was my being away from my family because of the cancer treatment. Wendy decided the best way to fix that problem was to create from her contacts a network of supporters who could reach out and let me know I was not alone. Her plan was no imposition to me, required little work on her own part, and always left me in control of what happened to me. It was years after my cancer treatment was over when I actually saw Wendy in the flesh again, and our friendship has been so enriched by her support for me in that time.

If thinkers have a flaw, it's that they can sometimes think too much. Whilst they are superb strategists and planners, thinkers can sometimes forget they are dealing with people, and not just problems. Thinkers tend to be pragmatists, and because they view complexities as challenges they don't always see the human being at the center of the issue. A great many health professionals are guilty of this because their primary motivation is to problem-solve the illness, and they may do this without considering the emotional or psychological needs of the patient. For thinkers, people are often defined by the problems they present, and a thinker may also presume their solution is not only welcome, but is the best one. Thinkers must take care to remain sensitive toward the person with cancer, and never merely impose their conclusions or plans upon them without consultation.

Your response to cancer is perfectly normal.

Mandy, Allie and Wendy all have very different personalities, strengths and weaknesses and past experiences, and thus had varying ways of dealing with a cancer diagnosis. Whether we're a doing kind of person, a deep feeler or a thinker, we all have our own default responses to crises. You may be like Mandy, interpreting news of a friend's cancer as a call to action. You may relate to Allie, and feel paralyzed by shock and sadness and unable to do a thing. You may find that like Wendy your mind goes into overdrive, creating ways to bridge gaps and solve problems. Each approach we take will bring its own benefits and advantages.

What sometimes isn't taken into account is how the person with cancer may feel or respond to whatever is said or done by others, or not said and done as the case may be. Those first few days and weeks can be a very strange, unsettled time. It's helpful to remember that because of this, gestures extended with the best of intentions can get a little lost in translation or even misunderstood completely. I haven't told you about the many things people did or didn't do which fell flat, offended me outright, or left me feeling neglected or intruded upon. The person with cancer might totally misinterpret something someone did or didn't for them for no other reason than they are simply having a bad day. They may misconstrue Allie's anxious silence as an attitude of cool indifference or as rudeness. They may see someone like Mandy as a control freak, or even accuse her of intruding. A person caught up in their own distress may even interpret thoughtful gestures like Wendy's with cynicism or sarcasm. We do, say and believe funny things when we're under stress, things we might not normally do, say or believe. A person who just found out they have cancer may be under a great deal of mental and emotional duress or quite ill, even in physical pain. This is a time to be very understanding - to have both thick and thin skin at the same time. We may have it in our head that people with cancer will always act with dignity and gratitude to our gestures, but that's an awful lot of pressure to be under when you're sick. If we retain the right to be upset and confused about their cancer, we will have to decide to extend that grace back to them and allow them to express all their own feelings about it as well, even if sometimes those feelings seem unreasonable or misdirected. People with cancer can become demanding and grumpy, and the whole thing can go on for months and years. This is probably going to get messy sometimes, and the fewer expectations you have of one another, particularly when it comes to good behavior and not hurting each others feelings, the better.

Whatever the circumstances and your own emotional state in the initial stages of your friend's cancer journey, remember in all likelihood none of it will stay the same very long. As more information comes to light, things will probably change. The way we behave at first is usually a simple reflex response to a perceived emergency, and in time, everything may settle down into some kind of rhythm. Finding your rhythm as a friend, carer for or

---

support person of for someone with cancer takes time. No matter how urgent this situation may feel at the outset, ease yourself into it. You may be there for quite a while.

Things to remember –

- *Your response to the situation will be shaded by your personality, your personal experiences and your feelings about the cancer and the person being diagnosed. There is no right or wrong way to react.*

- *Whatever your reflexive response to do, feel or think, you have a place in your loved ones cancer journey. Be mindful of your own motivations, and don't hesitate to seek support for yourself if you need it.*

- *A cancer journey is seldom easy for the people involved. Take your time to find your rhythm and don't overcommit yourself.*

- *Be gracious, compassionate and forgiving with both the person who has cancer, and with yourself. Now is not the time to have high expectations. Use this as an opportunity to learn about yourself and each other.*

- *While cancer may be the worst thing that has ever happened to your loved one, it doesn't have to be the worst thing that ever happened to your relationship. Where it is within your power, let it make and not break you. That way, cancer never, ever wins.* ☺

4

Settling Down With The Devil

Some things that might happen next to someone who has cancer.

So here we are a short time after the terrible news first broke. The initial crisis has passed, and the shock is beginning to abate. The cancer treatment prescribed for your friend or loved one may have already begun, and any side effects may be kicking in. Apart from all the things you may have expected, something else is happening you thought was impossible – you're starting to get used to the idea that someone you know has cancer.

Is this anything like you'd imagined it would be? Did it play out like a movie, or were there some surprises for you? Did people react the way you expected? Did *you* react the way you expected?

Now those first intense emotions surrounding the diagnosis have begun to subside, this is probably a good time for you as a carer or supporter to consolidate your thoughts and feelings, and perhaps spend some time thinking about what may be about to happen next.

There could be some big decisions ahead for your friend or loved one. They may be considering their treatment options, or perhaps even considering whether there are any options. This may mean they are scheduled for, or have already had, a barrage of tests, biopsies, scans and appointments. This is an anxious and frustrating time for the person with cancer, but it can be just as anxious and frustrating a time for the people around them.

Some things that happen when someone has cancer.

Many of these things will have already happened, but understanding what processes your loved one has already undergone will help you appreciate what they may be thinking and feeling in the first plateau phase after the crisis has abated.

Tests

Tests for cancer can vary from blood and pathology results, biopsies, scans and x-rays and surgery, and are used to locate, diagnose and stage cancer. Check the glossary at the back of this book for a basic explanation of many of the standard tests for cancer.

Staging.

Once the disease has been found and identified, it will be staged. Staging means deciding how advanced the cancer is. Staging is different between cancer types, but in general terms, stages progress from one through four - one being very early stages, and four meaning very advanced. There may then be a letter – either "A" or "B" – allocated to the staging number. "A" means that the cancer is still in its primary stages, and hasn't spread anywhere else, and "B" means that the cancer has begun to spread to or is found in other organs and tissues. Knowing this already will help when your friend tells you what stage cancer they have, because you can figure it out in your head without having to ask them what it all means, especially if they tell you they are a 3 or 4B.

Treatment options.

After tests and staging, next are discussions about treatment options such as surgery, chemotherapy and/or radiotherapy. These discussions may happen in a hurry or they may seem to drag on a bit while everyone makes up their mind. Don't read anything into this in terms of outcomes. In other words, don't panic.

Deciding on treatment options can be a difficult time. There may be side effects needing careful consideration, or logistics requiring complex planning. When it was decided I needed radiotherapy, it became clear I would have to spend two months staying in Sydney, close to the hospital where radiotherapy was available. This meant I would be four hundred kilometres away from home at a time when I needed my friends and family the most. It was a difficult decision to make, but we believed it was the right thing to do to give me the best possible chance of being cured. I found out later that given the choice, some young women with breast cancer chose to have more radical treatments such as mastectomy rather than leave their families for that amount of time. These kinds of choices are very personal, never easy and can have permanent ramifications, so where possible the people involved may take some time to work them out. It's important to be as nonjudgmental and understanding as possible. Have confidence your loved one will choose the option that is best for them, the one they feel they can deal with the best.

Thinking about alternatives – what's your role?

We all want the best for the person we love, and when they have cancer is no exception. You may find you disagree with their choice of a certain treatment, or you may even know of an option you consider to be superior. Be very careful about giving your opinion or advice about treatment choices you may think are a better option unless you are acting in a professional capacity and your services have been engaged. As a carer or supporter, it's more empowering and affirming to lend your support to their own well-informed choices. If they express frustration with the options they are being presented with, you may wish to offer to help them seek another opinion, but do not take your friends cancer to be an opportunity to present your personal beliefs about a particular therapy, treatment or health related product you heard about.

When I was having cancer treatment, I had two separate people buy and give me a copy of a very large, very expensive and very comprehensive cancer-curing diet book. I know they only wanted to help but a simple, open question along the lines of "What about alternative treatments?" would have saved them a lot of money. I had no intention of making such drastic changes to my lifestyle at that time as commencing an all-raw-food diet. I was eating a healthy variety of simple to prepare foods, and considering I was my own primary carer, that was more than enough for me to cope with. In the years since my own cancer, I have seen a great deal of financial strain and upset caused by people who felt it was necessary to use cancer as an opportunity to present their own particular views, product or agenda, or worse, to make money.

In the cancer support group I facilitated, the treatment options represented were as varied as the people using them. Some were taking the chemo/radio path, and others were juice-fasting, undertaking special diets or else taking various supplements to treat their cancer. We had a policy of not passing judgment on others choice of cancer treatment. Our group was a cancer-cure-evangelist-free zone. People were free to talk about the challenges and benefits of their particular treatment, but we would not accept any discussion around how one option was superior to another, allow any selling or advertising, or permit any criticism aimed at denigrating others treatment choices.

Carers, supporters, and even other cancer patients have a moral obligation to remain impartial when it comes to choices about therapies and treatment options. For me, one particular incident springs to mind, and I believe this is probably how I came to feel so strongly on the subject.

A few years ago, a lady from our church was diagnosed with very advanced bowel cancer. The pastor, an elder and I went to visit with Jenny and pray for her in the hospital. As soon as we entered the room, it was evident she was gravely ill. Jenny proclaimed she had decided not to acknowledge cancers power over her, and would take whatever treatment the doctors offered her to beat it. Jenny then shared with us some issues she was having with her two sons, issues which clearly needed to be resolved quickly in light of her failing health. Jenny was adamant she would not forgive her boys – there was plenty of time for them to come to their senses. It was clear to us Jenny was not ready to face the inevitability of her death. We prayed with her, but I suspected I would not see Jenny again.

Soon afterwards, I found out someone had told her about an "alternative" cancer clinic on the other side of the country getting "amazing results", but which cost a huge amount of money. Jenny told everyone she had changed her mind about the hospital treatment, and wanted to go to the clinic instead. She was still refusing to see her sons, or get her affairs in any kind of order. Despite having walked out of her retail business the day she was diagnosed, Jenny would not allow her assistant manager to take her place, believing if she could just get at that "treatment", she would be able to waltz back and into her life and pick up as if nothing had happened. Jenny's entire focus was now on getting herself out of the hospital and on a plane to the other side of the country. To my horror, I found out the person who told her about the clinic was a nurse who had been looking after her in the hospital.

My suspicions were right – I did not see Jenny again. She died less than two weeks later, still in the hospital.

After the funeral, Jenny's sons took the executor of the will to court for their share of the estate, because she never did make peace with them before she died. I walked past her business a month later, "closing down" signs now plastered across the windows. I grieved for this amazing, strong, talented mother and businesswoman who left this earth so consumed with a false hope she didn't even think to say goodbye to her children. I don't know if Jenny sent a cheque to that clinic, but I suspect if she did, they cashed it.

Jenny's situation also demonstrates how hard it can be to know what to do if your friend chooses something you morally or personally object to. I question the judgment of that particular nurse in suggesting such a thing to someone under her professional care. I remember Jenny's best friend telling us "What can I say? She's decided this is what she wants. Who am I to tell her she can't?" What a terrible position to be placed in. Surely it would have been wiser – and morally responsible - for that particular heath professional to support Jenny to a place of understanding the most important thing for her to do was attend to her affairs and make peace with her family, at least *before* she made plans to travel to an expensive clinic several thousand miles away.

If you suspect your loved one isn't satisfied by the answers they've been given by their health professional, or seems conflicted about the advice they have received, go back to your open questions and try to initiate a conversation around the subject. Perhaps Jenny's friend might have asked some exploratory questions. *What has happened to make you feel like the options here are now unsuitable? What will be solved by going to this clinic that cannot be solved by staying here? What's the most important thing to do right now, considering all the information you have about your current situation?* In opening up a discussion, she may have been able to help Jenny gain a deeper insight into the situation. Our role as her supporters was to help Jenny prioritize the things she needed and wanted to do based on the facts and information she knew to be true. Her death was inevitable, but did not need to be quite so traumatic for everyone involved.

Remember, as a supporter, you're not trying to guide the person to a particular conclusion. You're supporting them to consider all of their options, and make an informed decision. Above all, you're respecting their choices.

Let's say we're supporting a friend who's been told surgery is his only treatment option, but he is expressing reticence about the implications of this. A closed conversational approach might be, "It does sound drastic. Is surgery really necessary? You should get a second opinion from someone else." Another option might be, "Are you comfortable with the treatment choices you've been offered? Can I help you with what you want to do next?" The former approach infers that their doctor may not have their best interests at heart, and sows doubt in their mind regarding their own capacity to make a good decision. The latter approach however reinforces the idea that they have choices and can indeed make good ones, and also lets them know your motive is only to support both those ideas.

IMPORTANT - The exception to all this of course will be in cases where legal guardianship or power of attorney is in place over a patient. When a legal agreement has been made in advance regarding who has the right to make medical decisions for the patient, that agreement must be actively adhered to, and the patients wishes carried out by the person with the legal power to enforce them. But without a prior-standing legal agreement, the carers role and primary obligation is to support the cancer patient in their own choices. Please seek the advice of a social worker or legal advisor concerning power of attorney or legal guardianship.

Treatment that doesn't cure cancer.

While we always hope there is something we can do to cure cancer, there are times when the treatment offered isn't going to make cancer go away. Some kinds of treatment are given for reasons other than providing a cure. Treatment designed to alleviate the discomfort or pain of the cancer, but which it's known won't make cancer go away, is called "palliative treatment". However, when you hear the word "palliative", please do not presume your friend is going to die imminently. Palliative care can go on for some time, and will be planned across many stages with various contingencies considered and catered for. Palliative treatment is still cancer treatment, and is not "giving up". In the case of palliative cancer treatment, there will likely be many more bridges to cross and many wonderful times to be had before the time comes to say goodbye.

Sometimes it's very hard for cancer patients experiencing the palliative stages to talk to people about it. This can be because of the way people behave when they hear the word "palliative". A friend I once worked with in a survivorship program called this phenomena "coffin eyes" – the expression people often get on their faces when they realize the person right in front of them is very sick or dying. You first start noticing "coffin eyes" right after you find out you have cancer. At first, you don't understand, but then you work it out. The person you're talking to is playing a movie of your funeral in their head. They're imagining what it will be like to deliver your eulogy, and they're picturing themselves weeping at your graveside. They're wondering if the next time they hear your name mentioned is when it appears in the local newspaper under "death notices". The first few times you see "coffin eyes" it can be quite upsetting. Then it's funny. Then it just gets boring. Many people across various stages of cancer, palliative or otherwise, are walking around pretending everything is perfectly normal simply because they are trying to avoid ever seeing that dreadful expression on someone's face.

What most people don't realize is that if they begin to grieve a person who has cancer as if they already died, they will inadvertently speak and act differently toward them - and it will not be a happy kind of different. I used to think cancer support groups were for people who liked to sit around and whine about having cancer all day, but when I started a cancer support group, I discovered most of our time was spent talking about other quite fabulous and interesting things. Everyone couldn't wait to get to the meetings because it was one of the only places we could have conversations without looking at peoples "coffin eyes".

So you're having treatment – you're all better now, right?

For many people who have cancer, the treatment phase can make them feel much worse than the cancer. Often the disease itself causes no pain or discomfort, and the real sickness part kicks in as a side effect of treatment. This was certainly the case for me. I had few symptoms of cancer, other than feeling like I had the flu. I had no apparent lumps or bumps, and no obvious indication I had a very large tumour inside my chest. For me, the biopsies, scans, toxic chemicals and irradiation and all their various side effects were far more distressing and painful. I had a wire threaded into a vein through a small hole they punctured into the skin inside my elbow, so they could push a tube up past my shoulder and into my chest, and through this tube they gave me chemotherapy. The entry site for the tube became infected several times. Each biopsy – two in my chest, and one in my hip – involved someone pushing a foot-long needle through my flesh and into my bone and digging around with it. The chemotherapy made my hair fall out – *all my hair* – gave me mouth ulcers and caused my fingernails and toenails to crumble. One of my teeth broke off. I went into menopause. The radiotherapy gave me anemia and a very nasty case of shingles. In the end, I thought that dying of cancer might just be the least of my problems.

Friends and family members might expect once treatment commences the person with cancer will start to feel better right away. As a close supporter or carer, it's important to make yourself familiar with what treatment is going to be given and the possible side effects. As well as helping you know what to expect, this can also prevent embarrassing faux pas. One of the confusing side-effects of chemotherapy can be a ruddy, flushed complexion, so people would often say to me "Gosh, you look so well!" taking my tanned-looking face to mean my health was improving. Of the all the things people who have cancer tell me annoy them the most, being told they look fantastic when they feel shocking is one of the most common.

"I'd really like to see you."

From time to time when I was having treatment, I received phone calls and visits from people I didn't really know that well. I thought it was nice they showed an interest, but after a while it became clear they were not being supportive. *They were being investigative.* Not content to be informed via my close friends or family about my progress, they wanted to know exactly what was going on direct from the source. Sometimes I had the impression from people didn't want to see me so much as they wanted to *take a look at me.*

"How do you feel?"

As cancer patients, we don't always want to talk about how we feel. This is where open questions help quite a lot. If you ask how things are generally without specifically mentioning our health, if we want to talk about it we can. But if we'd rather not, we can always change the subject because you've given us the option to avoid it.

To help you perhaps understand why these last two points are such an issue, I tell you this. Your friend with cancer has been poked, prodded, stripped naked, had plastic tubes, needles and metal objects pushed into their body, had pictures taken of them from every possible angle, had those pictures discussed in front of them as if they weren't even in the room, and had their body talked about as if it were fifty pounds of interesting cheese. They might want to tell you about all this, but they could just as easily not want to talk about it any more, thank you very much. Perhaps they were happy to discuss it yesterday, but would rather just talk about anything else today. If in doubt, just ask them straight out, "Do you want to talk about how you feel?" They'll leave you in no doubt as to what they want to talk about.

Having cancer treatment, you come to understand what is really meant by "one day at a time". It's difficult to make plans. You don't know if you'll feel well from one day to the next. Some days you feel like facing people, and other days you don't. People treat you differently and you hate them for it – other days, people act like nothing has changed and that makes you crazy too. Cancer makes people do and say strange things sometimes, and sometimes the ones doing the strange things will be the person with the cancer. Sometimes it will be you as the carer or supporter. Remember – be gracious. Be honest and open about what's happening, and be compassionate for the times it doesn't go so well.

Things to remember –

- *The initial treatment phase of cancer can be filled with decision making and dealing with various side -effects. Learn to take things day by day and don't have high expectations during this time.*

- *Your role is to support their quest for answers and respect any choices they make about their treatment.*

- *Treatment can take some time to become fully effective, and side effects can cycle through the course of a regime.*

If you are involved in hands-on support or care, you'll need to remain flexible and keep an open mind

- *Use open questions when asking about their sense of well-being and allow them to have their bad days without feeling pressured to "be strong" or put on a brave face.*

- *Don't assume because they look "well", that they feel great too. Ask them "Do you want me to ask how you're feeling?" You'll soon find out if the topic is open for discussion.* ☺

5

The Role of Carer.
Finding your place in the cancer journey.

People say the darndest things when they're frightened, and few things shock us more than finding out someone we care for has been diagnosed with cancer. In the few years since I had cancer I've come to foster a greater appreciation for how others feel when faced with this kind of news, and what kinds of issues a diagnosis can bring up for friends and family. I've seen how those close to a person with cancer can become very anxious thinking about changes the cancer might bring, particularly in terms of what may be expected of them. These feelings are often hard to express because when someone is diagnosed with cancer, the last thing anyone wants to say is "But what about me?"

There are some common challenges supporters and carers face when making an emotional and/or physical commitment to caring for a person with cancer. The truth is, these issues are so complex and varied they warrant a whole book all of their own, and so we'll be merely identifying a few of the most common ones. I won't attempt to discuss all the challenges carers and supporters face in committing to the role, however I will attempt to normalize and validate some of the feelings we may face at the outset when considering taking on a formal caring role.

One of the hardest decisions we may ever have to make is deciding how involved to become when a friend or family member is diagnosed with cancer. Many factors must be considered – our relationship to the person, their actual needs and preferences, and our availability and any existing commitments we have. Naturally, everyone involved wants to help the best way they can, but exactly who does what isn't always clearly defined, and may not even be formally articulated. The most common offers a person with cancer will receive, particularly at first, are for meals, transport or housework, and these are seldom refused. But some of the more complex needs of a cancer patient require a deeper commitment from a carer or supporter. A formal primary caring role may simply fall to a particular person by default, or decisions may result from conversations and negotiations between the person with cancer and their friends, family and other support networks.

What is a carer?

In terms of formal supporting roles for a person with cancer, the one most commonly recognized is that of *carer*. As a term I've used already in this book, it's probably time we unpacked it. A carer is defined as someone who helps and supports a person through a disease or disability, in this case, cancer.[**] Carers may provide substantial physical and logistical support for the person,

---

[**] Cancer Council NSW, Understanding Cancer series, Caring For Someone With Cancer, page 4, Who Is A Carer? http://www.cancercouncil.com.au/685/cc-publications/understanding-cancer-series/cancer-carer/caring-for-someone-with-cancer-2/?pp=685

or they may only provide a basic level. The role of carer is not limited to the definition of one person or people providing physical, emotional or logistical support for another, there may be one primary carer, or caring can come from a team of people. Carers can be family members, friends, more distant relatives, perhaps even neighbors, or else professional or volunteer support workers. *Carer* literally means *one who cares,* so everyone who is involved emotionally or physically, or otherwise impacted by the cancer in some way, might be thought of as a carer. However, the label *carer* is usually reserved for a primary person assuming the role of companion or caregiver for the person receiving care.

One of the challenges facing supporters generally and particularly concerning carers is managing expectations and assumptions surrounding the assignment, acceptance and execution of caring responsibilities. If we're particularly close to the person diagnosed, before any arrangements are formally made one of the first things we may think about is how any anticipated changes may impact negatively on our own lives. These thoughts can be a source of shame and guilt for many people, and we might consider ourselves selfish for having them. They are however perfectly normal and understandable. Cancer can bring huge changes to everyone concerned, and even if the cancer goes away again, things don't always go back to normal. Any commitment to the person going through cancer and treatment on the part of family and friends needs to be very carefully considered.

Every case of cancer will require different levels of care and support. Any support required may fluctuate over the period of the illness and treatment, and provisions and tasks can also overlap between supporters. Things can become complex at times, and both deficits and surpluses can occur. It's absolutely possible to have too much lasagna brought to the door by well-meaning friends and neighbors, and it is not selfish for a cancer carer to feel they have been let down if others don't lend their support. After the initial emotion has subsided, the true implications of a supporting commitment can be difficult to maintain. Some may rush in with offers and quickly find themselves out of their depth, or even just bored. On the flip side, we might find ourselves pulling back from the person with cancer in the first instance because we're afraid too much will be expected of us. All these responses are common and natural, and anyone close to a person with cancer who has felt like this need not feel guilty or embarrassed. When situations like cancer arise, we all simply do the best we can, and with this in mind we need to keep our sense of humor and compassion for each other. Whilst we may succeed in normalizing cancer and the things that happen because of it to a certain degree, cancer inevitably brings up a wide variety of what can be very complex issues. These issues may sometimes prove more difficult to deal with than the cancer itself.

When it comes to the role of primary carer, this is sometimes formalized, but can also simply fall to a particular person for various reasons, as with my friend Lisa and her mother. Lisa's mother experienced some minor personality changes and after some tests was diagnosed with an aggressive – and incurable - brain tumor. Lisa found after her mother was diagnosed she simply 'became' her mothers carer without any arrangement being formally made, a situation Lisa partly attributes to her being the eldest of her siblings. But Lisa also describes becoming her mother's carer as " just a natural fit". The illness progressed quickly, and Lisa soon found herself not just supporting her mother with day-to-day tasks, but nursing her as well. Lisa treasures the last days they spent together, and believes she learned much about the process of death and dying by supporting her mother as she eased into the final chapter of her life. Lisa reflects on her experience as a carer with joy and satisfaction, and believes this period enriched both hers and her mothers life enormously.

Angie became a carer in quite different circumstances from Lisa. When Angie's sister-in-law and best friend Pam became ill with breast cancer, Angie stepped in as primary carer, supporting Pam physically and emotionally through the duration of her illness. Sadly, despite six and a half years of at times grueling treatment, single mother Pam died leaving her two children aged 17 and 21. Angie continued her role as carer by assuming mothering guardianship of Pam's children. Angie now works for a cancer charity, promoting the work of carers and facilitating support programs for cancer survivors. She speaks from her close and personal experience about the challenges carers face and the need for understanding about the role of carer in the cancer journey.

Angie took on a formidable task, supporting not just Pam but her family as well. This highlights the crucial importance of carers making their own well-being a priority. Spousal and platonic carers are often very similar in age to the person being diagnosed, and this can work for or against the situation. Pam's relatively young age made her passing especially sad, particularly in light of the two children she left behind, but because Angie too was in her forties at and in excellent health she was perhaps best placed to manage, albeit under considerable stress. However, with the majority of cancer diagnoses occurring over the age of fifty, we may safely assume most carers are also in this age group, and may even suffer health issues of their own. No wonder many carers can feel overwhelmed by the task ahead of them, and need some support as well.

Janice was in her late fifties, divorced, had stage-four lung cancer despite having never smoked, and was a truly formidable presence. She and her carer Beth came to the very first support group meeting I ever facilitated, and Janice warned me straight up that I better have a strong leadership style. Janice lived by the credo that if as a woman she was allocated twenty thousand words to utter each day, she was fully entitled to use up every one of them. Beth was a widow with two children who lived overseas, and when Janice lost her house around the same time as she was diagnosed, Beth invited her to move in. From the time their arrangement began until I met them eighteen months later they were virtually inseparable.

There was some inevitable small-town gossip about the nature of their relationship, against which Janice protected Beth fiercely. Beth in turn supported Janice with tireless care and meticulous organization, and wherever they went they arrived with something lovely to eat and something interesting to say. Their relationship, according to them, was purely a matter of practicality and convenience, but anyone who met them could see the true depth and sincerity of their regard for one another. Janice gave the air of being independent and in control, but in reality, without Beth, she simply would never have coped.

Janice passed away a few months ago, and for the first time it was evident just how tired Beth really was. I attended Janice's funeral and was shocked to see bustling, cheerful Beth shuffling along supported by two friends, both knees hobbled with arthritis. She looked completely exhausted. With Janice no longer striding two steps ahead of her keeping her going, Beth conceded it was her time to be on the receiving end of some care and attention. Theirs had been a very rare connection, and Beth would never accept suggestions what she did for Janice was in any way a sacrifice. However, caring for Janice had been a full-time job, and Beth had poured out the very best of herself in doing it.

We may always presume carers are either the peers or the elders of their charges, but this is certainly not always the case. Yesterday, my friend Maree and I were sharing a meal at her home. "I watched that little video clip you have on your website, " she remarked between mouthfuls, "and I wanted to tell you just how ungrateful you are." Even though she was half-joking, I was taken aback. A few months ago, I filmed a short montage of myself playing different characters, all stating a "thing not to say to someone who has cancer" to camera. One particular character I created popped up again and again, each time with another plate of lasagna in her hands. I was trying to light-heartedly demonstrate how a person with cancer can most certainly be given too many dishes of pasta bake by well-meaning friends. "I sure wish when my mother had cancer we had that problem," Maree explained. "I was ten when my mother had cancer, and I ended up being the one who looked after her. We ate a lot of spaghetti bolognese, because it was all I could cook. I sure wish I'd had your problem." I felt embarrassed, and spoiled. Maree had become her mothers' primary cancer carer at a very tender age, a role she carried on for three years until her mother passed away. Maree's situation highlights the fact that carers can be any age, and also demonstrates the need for all of us to be aware of the inadvertent and sometimes overwhelming roles close family and friends can be obliged to take on when someone is diagnosed with cancer.

However a carer comes to be one, the role can be incredibly rewarding, but also all consuming, often taking over a carers life completely. Many understand this at the outset and choose it anyway, however, many carers will feel obliged to assume the role and may feel unprepared and ill equipped, even resentful. Whether carers become carers by choice or by default, whether they cope well or feel overwhelmed, one thing I know about all of them -

Carers need as much support – physical, emotional and logistical - as the person they are caring for.

Caring for a person with cancer, particularly older or much younger carers, or those with existing health issues, can have serious and even irreversible implications for the persons' well-being. Every single carer needs others who will watch over them, provide respite where required and support them in taking good care of themselves. I have found it's quite common for a person who has been a long-term carer for a person with cancer to be diagnosed themselves with a serious illness not long after the subject of their caring has passed away.

With this in mind, it may well be that your particular role in a loved ones cancer journey won't be about providing them with direct support. Your energies may be better placed - and far more welcome - supporting their carer or carers.

The four stories I've highlighted above demonstrate how either family or friends of the person with the cancer can assume primary caring responsibilities, however, not everyone has a primary carer when they have cancer. This can be because nobody is available to fulfill the role, or because the situation itself does not sufficiently warrant it. When I was diagnosed I didn't have a primary carer in the technical sense, however various "caring" responsibilities were delegated and re-delegated amongst our family and friends in response to my illness. My husband took over from me as primary caregiver for our four children, whilst others stepped in to provide general support to all of us. Since I had cancer I've met many other people who didn't have a primary carer – and in some cases, as with Maree and her mother, not even a network of caring supporters - for various reasons.

Paul came along to our very first support meeting. A male breast cancer survivor, Paul presented with the façade of a tough old trooper, but it didn't take much prompting to reach the soft heart underneath. Paul told us all how relieved he was to find a group of compatriots, because his request to attend the local breast cancer support group had been declined on the basis of his gender - they'd never had to consider extending membership to a man before. Paul decided if they didn't want him, he didn't need them, and made himself a part of our general cancer support group instead.

A strong and resilient soul, Paul was able to cope emotionally after his diagnosis because of his firm will and independence. Apart from his adult son who lived in another city, Paul had no family to call on, lived alone, and had few of the kinds of friends who could step in to help him emotionally or even practically. Paul seemed lonely, and was often confused by the virility of his own emotions, the strongest of which was anger. Paul was angry at the breast cancer support group who rejected him, angry at his specialist for being flippant when presenting his treatment options, and angry about the lack of services for men with breast cancer. Coming to our support group helped to meet his need for empathic support and understanding, but Paul knew he was pretty much doing it alone. The nature of his cancer was already emasculating, and this, coupled with his fierce need for independence, made for a tough, lonely journey through cancer. True to form, Paul had us all believing he didn't want it any other way.

Because cancer can provoke very strong emotional responses in different people, it can be difficult for friends and family to work out where exactly they fit into the picture. As I mentioned previously, a cancer diagnosis does not always cause people to draw closer. Sometimes even the closest family members may feel repelled, and they may be as confused by their actions as the person with the cancer. To add further complexity, if a relationship was strained or ambivalent before the cancer came along, any issues arising from the illness can present a real test, and the results can sometimes decide the relationship once and for all.

When I was in Sydney having radiotherapy, I met Tracey, also having treatment but for breast cancer. A single mother from a country town, Tracey left her daughter to stay at home with Tracey's father, long since divorced from her mother. Before her diagnosis Tracey and her mother were tentatively working through some long-standing issues with their relationship, but this had come to a halt around the time Tracey had surgery. Strangely, Tracey's mother hadn't contacted her since her hospitalization, and despite the fact she lived in the same city where Tracey was having radiotherapy, hadn't come to visit and didn't answer her phone. Tracey discovered her mother was holidaying on an ocean cruise and wouldn't be back until long after Tracey finished treatment. Despite the fact they weren't especially close before the diagnosis and her mothers holiday had probably been planned for quite some time prior, Tracey felt abandoned, physically and emotionally. She wondered if their relationship could ever reconcile to a point where Tracey could articulate to her mother how hurt she felt by her distance and apparent indifference to this difficult time in her daughters life.

What happened between Tracey and her mother is one example of how unspoken expectations can create problems between a person with cancer and the people around them. We may expect certain people will play particular roles in our cancer story, as Tracey did with her mother, perhaps not unreasonably. Relationships can shift drastically as roles change and dependencies shift. For example, someone who is normally physically and emotionally independent may suddenly feel vulnerable and needy. But a cancer diagnosis doesn't always make a person feel disempowered and vulnerable. Many people find they become stronger and more self-assured, and may surprise the people around them with their stoicism and independence. Someone who offers their help or support may be rebuffed or rejected. Obviously, this too can cause problems,

Don't assume the worst.

Just because they've been diagnosed with cancer, no need to act as if your friend of loved one is going to die soon. This is important because believing someone we love is dying will definitely change the way we behave and speak when we're with them, and may even have us promising them the world when we are unable to deliver it. Even if the prognosis isn't particularly good, their lives may not change at least in the interim as much as we think. They may not feel anywhere near as bad as you expect, and they may be less distressed and concerned about their having cancer than you are.

Don't be a hero.

Caught up in the emotion of finding out the person has cancer, many people rush in with grand offers of help at the beginning they realize later were too much for them to keep up. Before you leap in, be mindful of your predisposition to instinctively *do, feel or think.* Consider carefully what you're able to commit to. If you are likely to become a primary carer, be realistic about what are likely to be your shortcomings, and seek help and support for yourself as well as the person you'll be caring for.

Warm shoulders are much nicer than cold ones.

The thought of being obliged or expected to help may absolutely terrify us. The emotional turmoil a cancer diagnosis can bring may simply feel like too much to bear and may make you want to pull away. A situation like cancer which you can't control and aren't able to fix may even be quite repellent. Our instinct when we feel we lack the capacity to cope may be to step away from the situation, to be cool, or even to diminish the seriousness of it. Your emotions may be confusing or confronting to you, and you might not even understand them, but these are natural reactions, a defense mechanism to protect us from being hurt. When I had cancer, I was surprised to find some of the people I thought would be available to me pulled away, while others out on the peripherals drew closer. People for whom my having cancer was really none of their business became my very close friends, whilst others I'd been intimate with drifted out of my life altogether. By the time my health had improved, for one of my closest friendships in particular, too much water had passed under the bridge. I can't help feeling this particular friends' brusque attitude towards me came more from a sense of their own fear of failing me than any actual expectation I'd had of them. I would've been satisfied with a warm shoulder to lean on and a friendly conversation from time to time, if it had meant holding onto the friendship. Those interactions can be painful, but surely are worth it.

Take time out.

Even a full-time, live in carer must have some respite from time to time. You must get sufficient rest, adequate nutrition and have some kind of life away from the person with cancer. This is a normal part of any functional, mature relationship, and caring for a sick person is no exception. There is a danger, particularly for long-term carers, of losing some perspective on life generally, and the isolating nature of the caring role can feed into this. I have seen carers become quite codependent on the person with the cancer where their whole identity is wrapped up in their ability to provide care for a person with cancer. In extreme cases carers foster an environment where the person with the cancer stays dependent on them long after the physical disease no longer warrants it, or deflect any attempts by others to provide care for either or both of them - defending their "turf". Carers need to be mindful of their social and mental health as well as nurturing their physical well being, particularly if the caring role is especially intense or long in duration.

Being a carer or close supporter of a person with cancer is a huge consideration, and must never be taken lightly. Each situation has it's own complexities and as such there are no hard and fast rules about taking on the role of carer. I suggest you sit down with the person who requires the caring and, carefully considering all factors, negotiate the role with them. Don't presume you as a carer are an island. Speak to the social worker attached to the patients' oncology unit, speak to your own doctor, and if necessary, ask for a referral to a counselor. There are support groups in existence catering exclusively for carers, and I strongly recommend seeking one out. It may help to attend a support group with the person who has cancer, but I see many carers in support groups reducing themselves to a shadow of the person with the cancer, placing all their own thoughts and feelings second in line. Let's face it – cancer is terrible, but cancer is not the worst thing that can happen to a person, and it will behoove us all to keep a sense of humor and perspective about it. I often wonder if there is not a second kind of "dying of cancer"…one where the selfless, humble carer is slowly dissolved and absorbed into the world of the person they are caring for, never to be seen or heard from again. Surely we must never tire in seeking a cure for that terrible demise as well.

Things to remember -

- *A carer can be anyone affected by the cancer, but usually means the person or persons providing primary or essential personal care for a person with cancer.*

- *Not everyone has, wants or needs a carer.*

- *Being close to a person with cancer can make some people feel like they want to jump in and help and others feel overwhelmed and repelled. Both responses are natural and nothing to be ashamed of.*

- *Those who wish to help a person with cancer may be better placed supporting the carer than the person with cancer, as this is often the greater need.*

- *Nobody gives out medals to carers. If you are considering becoming one, your own health and well-being must remain one of your highest priorities.*

- *When it comes to being a carer, remember...there is more than one way to die of cancer. Don't allow your self and identity to become absorbed by the illness of your loved one. They will benefit only if you are strong, supported and healthy in mind and body.* ☺

6

"What The Hell Is That About?"
When a person with cancer doesn't behave as you expect.

Most of the conversations I have on the subject of cancer are with
people worried about what they should say when they see their
friend for the first time after a diagnosis. However, some people I
talk to just want to know why their friend with cancer is acting so
strangely, weeks, or even months later. "They've changed," they
say, "and why did they slam the door in my face when I went
around to visit?" While a good many people appear to sail right
through cancer and treatment without too much trouble, some
seem to be constantly verging on a breakdown. Others behave as if
they're downright furious. We might turn up at their home with a
meal or a gift expecting a smile and a "Your help is much
appreciated, thank you very much!" to be told in no uncertain
terms *"Your help is not needed right now, thank you very much."*
We might try deliberately not to talk about cancer in their presence
only to be accused of being insensitive, or else work hard to create
open conversations only to be told we're intruding. Why do some
people act so weird when they have cancer? And why do others
behave as if everything is totally fine when they're actually
supposed to be so awfully sick?

A couple of years ago, I received an email from a friend,

concerned that a lady from their church wasn't handling having cancer very well. She wrote:

"Dear Jo, I have a question to ask.

"I have a good friend recently diagnosed with breast cancer, and I'm worried because I think she's behaving a little strangely. While she is part of a close-knit church community and seems to have quite a few friends, she hasn't told very many people that she has an advanced case of cancer - maybe five of us know how bad things are at the most. She's having chemotherapy at the moment, but she drives herself to treatment and doesn't want anyone to go with her. Being one of the few who know the truth, I feel deeply obliged to help her, but I live forty minutes drive away from her home so I can't do as much as I'd like to. Other people from our church congregation ask me about her all the time, but I don't feel I can say because she specifically asked me not to tell others about the gravity of her illness. She has four children whom she home-schools and they seem to be struggling behaviorally, but she shields them and won't let us take them away from her even just so she can have a rest.

"Whilst I respect her decision not to share her experiences with everyone because they might not share her beliefs and approve of her choices, her withholding from the other people at church who want to help has created a barrier between her and them. Now, people aren't bothering to ask after her because they know they won't find anything out. At the same time, she is angry because

91

people seem to have forgotten about her. Her belief is that people should continue to pray, provide support and bring meals without necessarily knowing why she needs them to. Like I said, I fully respect her decisions, knowing she is trying to stop people from gossiping and also protect her children from other people's emotional reactions. But is this aloof and distancing behavior normal?"

I'll show you my response to my friends' letter a little later, but suffice to say, this is a clear example of how sometimes the people who are trying to support a person with cancer can become very confused by the mixed signals they appear to send out. Is there some kind of code to follow? Are there rules? How can I be sure I don't offend or upset my friend when I offer them my help? Are they not obliged to accept everyone's help when it's offered so generously?

Why are they acting like this when I'm only trying to be nice?

Unfortunately, there is no code, and there are no rules. There are only *people* – fleshy, feeling, fumbling people, all of us with all our expectations, good intentions and limitations. We're all intent on simply doing our best, and we all want the same thing – for the person with cancer to be okay.

You have cancer, and I'm going to help you, dammit.

When you have cancer, it can feel like you have a huge obligation to behave in a particular way. You learn that people expect certain things of you, but nobody really tells you straight out what these things are. It seems there is a set of rather ambiguous societal rules for the ill and infirm, and any breaking of those rules can leave people questioning their good manners, mental health, or even make the well-intentioned suspicious about whether the person is really as "sick" as they claim to be.

A cancer diagnosis can create a subtle shift in the perceptions of others. No matter how marvelous or dreadful we were before we had cancer, no matter how philanthropic or selfish or humble or successful, people with cancer can find themselves suddenly treated as if we just won the grand final of Cancer Idol. Nothing we did, said or were before now matters one bit, in fact, people sometimes act as if everything we ever did before in our lives only ever lead up to this time. We're now the proud, unwitting owner of a sparkling new career as an inspirational Cancer Hero.

And like all celebrities, Cancer Heroes must make certain sacrifices. In exchange for the attention and adoration, the sympathy, the fear and the lasagna, we must pay. And often, just like garden-variety famous people, it's with our privacy and our freedom to choose.

Now this can be absolutely terrific, and can really work out well for all involved, provided everyone understands the boundaries and has their wants and needs met in the end. I really love those domestic make-over reality shows where someone with cancer has their house renovated. It's great when they're able to stand up at the end gazing at their practically brand-new house gratefully hugging their tearful family because about ten thousand "things-to-do-around-the-house" have just been just crossed off their list. Now they can simply focus on the matter at hand. But these folks, and their families and friends, pay a huge price – not necessarily financially, but in terms of their privacy and their personal identity, and this happens to a lesser degree to most people who are diagnosed with cancer. How do you ever do anything as impressive again in your life? How can anything ever compare to being a "cancer celebrity"? Managing the influence and impact of cancer on our lives can become a kind of complicated public relations exercise.

Cancer charities and organizations often use the "cancer celebrity" phenomena to their advantage, and I've personally been involved in several advertising and marketing campaigns designed to raise money for cancer research and support. In fact, when I was just a few months into my chemotherapy I agreed to have my photo taken for the local paper to help promote a popular cancer fundraiser. When I have spoken at cancer conferences and functions, I've always told my audience using my own experience as a way to raise money and awareness was how I "made cancer pay". As far as I was concerned, cancer took away part of my identity when it came to visit me, but it was no free ride. I was happy to use my "Cancer Idol" win and use that myth of the "cancer celebrity", if it meant we'd be growing closer to finding a cure, once and for all.

Changing the way we see someone just because they have cancer often happens because of the language we use when we talk about it. It goes back to the ideas we've already discussed – to the battle scenario and the war imagery. As well as being a kind of hero worship, cancer is also tied to the image of the "cancer victim". Ironically, much of the same things are expected from both celebrities and victims. Both must surrender a certain degree of privacy, and also, a certain degree of choice. A cancer diagnosis causes a subtle shift in power to occur, with the effect of limiting a person, while at the same time elevating them. It can be incredibly confusing as a person with cancer to be venerated as a kind of super-hero, while at the same time expected to surrender ones dignity and accept what essentially equates to charity.

Reading and sending out signals

When someone we care about has cancer, it can be very difficult to ask straight out exactly what they want us to do for them, if anything. It's usually much easier to look for subtle signals. However, this can cause problems. One person may decide that a certain set of circumstances, perhaps simply the cancer diagnosis itself, is a clear signal for them to get busy and do something, even if they haven't been specifically approached. This is perfectly understandable, and in most cases, if the gesture is carefully thought out and respectfully carried through, will be gratefully received. However, if the person with cancer was not aware they sent out such a signal, or does not want or need the gesture being extended, this can clearly cause all kinds of problems.

This issue of unspoken, inadvertent signals first became apparent to me when I was having treatment. Resting at home between chemotherapy treatments, it became clear the expectation amongst most people was I up for visitors anytime it was convenient for someone to drop by. However, I didn't always want a visitor, and it wasn't always convenient. Also, because the chemo compromised my immune system, I needed to reduce any risk of picking up viruses. But despite the fact we told our friends to call first, certain people continued to drop in whenever it was convenient for them. One didn't even knock but just walked right in and prowled around the house until they found me napping (and drooling unattractively). We needed a strong signal people would acknowledge. I made a sign and it taped to our front door explaining I was between cancer treatments, had a suppressed immune system, needed to rest and couldn't have visitors right now. It was a good plan and stopped unnecessary visits immediately.

This issue of mixed signals can become a real problem for people, as with my friend who wrote asking my advice. The ladies from church interpreted the woman's breast cancer as a signal for them to intervene, which was wonderful and absolutely appropriate. However, they misinterpreted the signal of her emotional withdrawal as her being recalcitrant, and thus viewed her refusal to divulge intimate details of the illness as gross rudeness. Their help was wanted and in all probability greatly appreciated, but what was not appreciated was their expectation she should surrender her dignity and privacy in return. These misread signals and unspoken assumptions almost caused a woman in need to be abandoned by the people she needed the most, and this whole misunderstanding could have been solved with empathic, open conversations between all concerned.

Most of the problems between people with cancer and their friends and family usually turn out to be unspoken, unrealistic or unrealized expectations of one another. Whenever someone expects another to do something or be something, and they don't or can't, this inevitably causes disappointment and confusion. Given also that cancer is such an emotional issue, people often come to it with their hearts beating right out on their sleeve. Protecting your personal boundaries as a cancer patient can be very, very tricky when people are being so incredibly nice, and want to help so very, very much.

But not everyone's expectations are around what they'd like to do for you. Some people have very definite ideas of how a person with cancer ought to behave, and don't mind letting you know what they are.

You don't act like a person who has cancer.

Not long after I started chemotherapy my husband and I were invited to lunch with some friends. I'd lost all my hair and quite a lot of weight, but my appetite for food and drink – in particular, for alcohol - was (at that time) perfectly fine. I remember picking up a bottle of red wine and eagerly pouring myself a glass just as we were sitting down to eat. Red wine had become one of my little occasional indulgences. One of my friends stopped in his tracks a few feet away from me, and stood there watching as I slurped at my wine before raising his eyebrows and acidly remarking "I see having cancer hasn't affected your ability to knock back a drink." I laughed, but he did not. He seemed quite offended by my behavior. Was I committing some terrible social faux pas by enjoying a glass of cabernet sauvignon over lunch with my friends and having cancer at the same time? My friends' husband clearly had his own ideas about how a person with cancer ought to behave - certainly as far as alcohol consumption was concerned. Apparently I just wasn't with his program.

You don't look like a person who has cancer.

We've all seen exactly what a person with cancer is supposed to look like. Pale, with dark circles under the eyes. Thin and emaciated. Head swathed in a scarf, bad wig, or else completely bald. You probably think you could tell a person with cancer from everyone else in a crowd. But you probably couldn't.

The fact is, not all people who have cancer look unwell, are painfully thin or even bald. As I've said, not everyone who has cancer loses their hair, and not everyone even gets particularly sick. Cancer is not just one disease – it's a plethora of diseases

---

98

with a vast number of symptoms, and even the treatment can have a wide variety of side effects, each of which affects different people in different ways. The same cancer can affect different people in various ways. Some people are walking around with cancer and you won't know until they tell you. I've met people who were dying of metastatic cancer who looked perfectly fine, and others with a cancer the size of a pimple who looked like death warmed over. Never. Make. Assumptions.

In the same way as cancer and treatment affect people in various ways, some people cope better with their cancer experience than others. Some will be devastated by it, but others may see the same disease or treatment as a minor nuisance. Some are angry, and others are indifferent. Some are not brave, and a good many adamantly refuse to "stay positive". Some of the most fun folks to be with I've met along my cancer journey were the ones who refused to be upbeat all the time. But some people find this awkward and confronting. A great friend of mine has a fantastic story about how she lost her prosthetic breast whilst surfing one day. When she told me the story for the first time, we roared with laughter. But she can't tell that story to just anyone, because she's found there are people who just don't find it one bit funny. "That's terrible. How can you be so flippant?" they will say. Rather than treating cancer as if talking about it will make it cross, many people with cancer choose instead to have some fun and laugh at it.

There's no need to be like that - I'm only trying to help.

———

The same friend tells me how one particular day she was at home waiting for her doctor to call her with some test results - results which would determine if she needed to go back and have her other breast removed, and a bit more of the most horrendous chemotherapy known to modern science. Her anxiety levels were peaking. Suddenly, there was a knock at the door, and when she opened it she found the mother of one of her daughters school friends standing on her doorstep. She had brought a small gift, would she like a visitor? My friend was startled and far too upset to entertain a guest, so she apologized and explained it was not a terribly good time before closing the door. Later that day, to her relief, her doctor called through with the results - everything was clear and no further treatment was needed.

A few days later my friend was walking from her home to the beach when she happened to see the lady who had knocked on the door earlier in the week walking toward her. As she grew closer, my friend made herself ready to explain why she hadn't been able to let her in, and apologize for her abruptness. She never had a chance to speak. The woman marched up to her and, with her finger pointed in her face, started yelling about what an impolite individual she was. She had never been treated like that in her life. *All I wanted to do was help. How could you be rude?* Shocked and in tears, my friend went straight home. Clearly, there were sincere good intentions on the part of her visitor, but there were also intense emotions and high expectations involved, however, under the circumstances she provided my friend no recourse but to deflect her good intentions. With the woman's feelings so badly hurt, and no allowance extended to my friend to explain herself, there was really no way to recover the friendship from such a terrible beginning.

I didn't think it would be like this.

As far as the letter from my friend at the beginning of this chapter is concerned, I took some time to consider my reply. I totally understood where she was coming from, genuinely confused as she was about who exactly was acting inappropriately. Was it her friend with the cancer? Or was it the group of would-be helpers from church? Which of them was making unfair demands of the other? Was it reasonable of the woman to expect the church ladies to drive for an hour each way to visit her, bringing hot food and praying the rest of the time for her healing, when they didn't even know exactly how bad the cancer was? Was it unfair for the church ladies to expect to know the woman's' private business just because she was a single mother with cancer who needed their help?

I replied:

"I think your friends response to the church ladies objections is reasonable, normal and in many ways very wise. I have found a few people, usually who never had cancer themselves, will have some fairly strong ideas about what will happen when someone has cancer. Some folks occasionally think it's their personal responsibility to make sure a person who has cancer is doing what they ought to do, and how they must behave. No wonder your friend doesn't want to tell many people what she's going through. She realizes that in one hot minute she would have far more of other people's opinions, judgments, advice and 'kind words' than she knows she can handle right now.

"As a community of Christians, are you and your friends not commissioned to help when a member of the church body needs it? I wonder then, why do some people apparently believe sick or very damaged people requiring help are a kind of 'public property'? They bring a hot meal to a sick mother, so they presume to have the right to know all her business as if being unwell means she must surrender her right to privacy. I'm afraid that I agree with your friend with the cancer – it sounds like she has some healthy personal boundaries. I think the church should continue to uphold her in prayer and bring her meals just as she's asked, and try and resist the temptation to make her purchase these services by satisfying the curiosity of her helpers. Their motives I'm sure are charitable, but surely they don't need to be rewarded for their good works by having your friend surrender her dignity.

"The last thing she needs to worry about is whether her church friends feelings are being hurt because she doesn't want to talk about having cancer. She is not worried about their feelings. She is worried about a future for her children, and wondering whether it will include their mother.

"I think this lady ought to extend her reach for support. Sometimes it's better to leave your friends out of it, because they may be too close to the situation to help. Please consider asking her if she would like some help from a community agency or charity organization. There are many service agencies I'm sure would be able to provide a housework service and support her with meals, perhaps even provide money to help with her bills.

"Your church has a wonderful opportunity to show true charity and grace by loving this mother and supporting her, no matter whether she 'plays ball' and acts like they think a person with cancer ought to. Tell those women start making casseroles. If they can't bake for her, for goodness sake, ask them to keep on praying!"

Things to remember -

- *What expectations might you have right now of your friend or family member? Are you set in your thinking about how what kinds of behavior they ought or are expected to exhibit simply because they have cancer? Do you think they should now behave and speak in a certain way?*

- *Is it likely you will change your opinion of them or the nature or severity of their illness if they upset, surprise or offend you with something they say or do? Don't assume your friend feels a certain way or wants a particular thing just because you thought all people with cancer felt and wanted those things.*

- *Make contact before visits to check if it's a good time to avoid setting both of you up for disappointments. Have you discussed the nature of your contact with them? Can you just drop in anytime? If you don't know them well enough to have this conversation, assume you always need to call first, and decide you won't take offense if they say no.*

- *All prior certainties between you may now be up for negotiation. All previous rules and boundaries between you might require clarification. Ask before you do things for or with your friend now, even if you've done those things for or with them every week for the past thirty years. Nothing may have changed, but don't assume anything.*

- *Take the pressure off both of you - don't expect your friend to be a sweet little saint at this time. They will be grumpy, rude and selfish sometimes. If they seem self-obsessed, don't worry. It probably won't last forever.*

- *Before you offer help or support to your friend or loved one with cancer, have a think about what your expectations are. If you go ahead and do what you plan, do they have any choice on how they may respond? Your motives may be totally pure, but if your gesture or action reduces the amount of options they have, including the option to say no thank you, you may need to revise your plan.*

- *In all your actions and words, make it a primary objective to always allow the object of your good intentions to retain their dignity and pride. They have a right to privacy and autonomy, and they may wish to retain it whilst also being in receipt of your goodwill. Don't make someone your "project". They'll be able to tell, trust me.*

- *How will you feel if they accept your hot meal, but don't make you a part of their "inner circle" of friends or visitors? If you see them smoking, eating fatty foods or drinking alcohol, will you feel differently about them? Most of the expectations we have of others set us up for disappointment, and the people we love who have cancer will be no exception. When offering support and practical assistance to someone with cancer, a helpful rule to abide by is no strings attached – no offense taken.*

- *Expecting someone to behave, respond or react in a certain way simply because they have cancer is setting you both up for disappointment. This is a good opportunity for you to challenge some of your assumptions and examine your presuppositions about cancer, and perhaps even learn some new ones.* ☺

7

The Fight, the Battle, and Other Redundant Cancer Phrases.
Why we all get to choose our own cancer adventure.

When I was diagnosed with cancer, I heard the word "fight" used right from the beginning. *You have to fight this, you're a fighter* and *we're all fighting right along with you* were things people said to me often. I certainly had a lot to fight for. My husband needed me - our four children were then aged 15, 11, 9 and 3 years old. At the age of 33, I still had so many things I wanted to do with my life. I was passionate about wanting to survive cancer and confident I could do it. I was all primed and ready for some cancer-fighting action.

If this is a battle, when do we start fighting?

But quite soon after my cancer diagnosis, far from feeling like some kind of warrior, I actually found I felt tired much of the time. Even though we now knew what was wrong with me, we really had no idea what was going to happen next. Would the treatment be painful? Would it make me even sicker? Was I going to die after all this and leave my husband to raise our children alone? Amongst all the apprehension and trauma I felt profoundly powerless, and despite my expectation that I'd be participating in my cancer healing somehow, I felt I wasn't actually doing anything to contribute to my getting better. Instead of doing any

7

real *cancer fighting*, there seemed to be just a lot of waiting around. I waited in waiting rooms for appointments. I waited for tests results. I waited for buses, cars and taxis to take me somewhere for more treatment and more results. I waited on puffy recliner chairs while toxic chemicals went down tubes into my arm. I waited for side effects to kick in and then abate again. And for six weeks, I waited every weekday morning at 10am to be ushered into a room and have radiation shot into my chest for ten seconds at a time, then waited for twenty-three hours until it was time to go back and do it again.

I grew frustrated. *I wanted me some good, proper cancer-battling action.* I wanted control. I wanted to get at this thing inside my body – this unseen blob that was trying to kill me – and rip it apart, attacking it with everything I had, physically, emotionally and mentally. But I couldn't. It was in there, buried in my chest, out of sight and out of reach. Besides, I didn't feel like going to war, I felt like going to bed. Having cancer was not anywhere as exciting as I'd hoped, and I didn't feel any more motivated as the months wore on. It was boring, tiring and repetitive. Others around me grew bored of it as well. This was nothing like the battle I'd expected. As the process of diagnosis, treatment and management progressed I began to see that there was probably not going to be many opportunities to do what I thought it meant to be *fighting cancer*.

When my treatment started, I tried imagining my chemotherapy to be little soldiers in my bloodstream running around shooting cancer cells, but it provided me with little comfort. How could I know the treatment was doing its job? Did my thinking "positive" even make a difference? I'd thought "fighting" would feel like *doing something to help get rid of the cancer*, but I didn't feel like I was doing anything at all. I felt passive and weak. Not only was my body being sabotaged by rampaging cancer cells, my whole life had been wrenched off course. I was now careening along a path I very much didn't want to go down. I felt cheated both by the fact that I had cancer and was probably going to die of it, and by the fact I'd been led to believe that I could somehow help stop it from happening by having a combative mental attitude. The truth was that for much of the time I didn't feel brave, strong or noble. I felt sad, sore and sorry for myself. I felt vulnerable and disempowered. I felt like every day I was just putting another one behind me. Most of the time I was simply obliged to accept what was happening, allowing everyone else to do whatever they wanted to me while I lay back and thought about something else. If I fought anything, it was the urge to tell people to just back off and leave me alone. I resented being seen as weak and needy, and I hated myself for being cranky at people when they only wanted to help. With all the lying around and the waiting for something to happen and the trying not to get angry at people, I soon began to think that learning to relax and be patient was probably going to do me a lot more good than fighting was.

For me, the cancer battle analogy seemed far more confusing than it was clarifying. No matter how ready I'd felt for a battle, no opportunity ever came for me to face-off with cancer. And rather than being brave, far more often I simply had to be *compliant*. I started to think the kind of courage cancer patients really had was nothing to do with fortitude or strength, but really had more to do with how prepared you were to let someone do painful, horrible and invasive things to your body without your slapping them in the face. In the end, "brave" seemed to me to just be something kind people said to people who had cancer to make them feel less passive, useless and redundant.

I certainly suffered as a result of the cancer both physically and emotionally, but "fighting" – which to me meant mental resistance, displays of stoicism and militant positive thinking – didn't turn out to be an effective mental strategy to manage either the stress or distress I was feeling. The image of putting one day behind me and beginning a new one seemed to help much more. I began to think of my cancer experience as more like a long, tedious walk with a destination at the end. On the news, I'd seen stories of people who raised money for charity by walking from one side of the country to the other. After enduring months of repetitive treatments, many of which made me feel battered and exhausted, and which never really seemed to get me anywhere, I felt I knew just how they felt. Every day they were closer to their goal, but every day was just the same as yesterday. Their progress across the land was a succession of steps, each one identical to the last. In my mind, cancer was a journey like that - a long, boring walk from one part of my life to another, a necessary toil to be tolerated and then be done with. I imagined a swimmer training by lapping endlessly up and down a pool, tumble-turning at each end and launching off to stroke yet another identical lap, growing stronger and more graceful with each lap. These mental pictures helped me far more than the fighting image ever did, and I still resist the battle metaphor when describing cancer to this day.

Finding our own metaphor.

Since that time, I've learned that a great many people with cancer are, unlike me, actually helped by the idea of fighting in a battle, and finding it hugely empowering and comforting. But then I found just as many who didn't appreciate the war metaphor at all. I became interested in learning how different people with varying life experiences and perspectives were able to integrate and process what was happening to them throughout their cancer experience. Through telling my own story, I was privy to the stories of many others, and I came to see that there are as many ways to define a cancer experience as there are ways to journey through it.

Through my roles in cancer supportive care, and learning how many cancer organizations view their role in combatting cancer through research and prevention, my own fiercely negative views on the "cancer battle" metaphor came to be tempered a little. I now believe that it is very important for each person to define, name and describe their own cancer experience in the language, and with the metaphors, that suit them the best.

There's more than one way to fight cancer.

Lynn was a formidable personality. Her strong Scottish accent coupled with her sturdy, square shouldered frame created the impression this was a woman not to be messed with. The ovarian cancer she was diagnosed with was in remission when she started coming along to our support group. We facilitated discussion around our circle by allowing each participant a few minutes speaking time, during which we re-introduced ourselves to any new members and updated our stories. Lynn loved to tell us how she lay in the recliner chair during her chemotherapy treatments, closing her eyes and imagining the toxic chemical "soldiers" rampaging through her bloodstream "taking out" any rogue cancer cells they happened across with their little machine guns. She firmly believed this helped her recover from cancer, and it provided comfort for her when she feared it might return. Iris, another support group member, had also had ovarian cancer, and related how she still had a pair of boxing gloves tied to the end of her bed. "It won't get me lying down!" she laughed. Unlike me, both Lynn and Iris found the empowering imagery of fighting a battle helpful mentally and emotionally. But there are other ways we can fight cancer as well.

Not long after I started treatment I became involved in volunteering for the Cancer Council, beginning a supportive relationship that continues to this day. The first time they asked me to help was by inviting me to have my photograph taken to accompany a media release for a local newspaper for Daffodil Day, a fundraising event where volunteers sell daffodils to raise money for cancer research and support services. Soon after I went into remission, the Cancer Council asked if I'd like to help them launch a new printed resource they'd produced to assist parents to talk to their children about cancer. Soon after that, I was invited to attend some training for a new initiative they were testing – *cancer consumer advocacy*. I learned that "cancer consumers" is a more empowering phrase cancer clinical services and support agencies often use to describe cancer patients, and advocacy means "speaking up in the place of". The Cancer Council trains cancer survivors to lobby governments and clinical/supportive care bodies for improvement to cancer services, increasing access to treatments, seeking approval to funding for research and promoting prevention programs. As a trained cancer advocate, I became involved in many different campaigns, with the strategic goal of helping people with cancer gain better access to treatment and support services. We lobbied a health service in one regional area to employ another oncologist at their hospital, which cut down the waiting times for cancer patients needing chemotherapy, some of whom had been waiting six weeks from their diagnosis to commence treatment. Another campaign focused on increasing government funding to my local hospital to purchase two radiotherapy machines, preventing cancer patients needing to travel to Sydney for extended periods for treatment, as I had been forced to do. This advocacy work, whilst time-consuming, was extremely gratifying, and advocates could see the lives of other cancer patients being improved in tangible ways because of our efforts. In attending meetings, designing campaigns and speaking to bureaucrats and politicians I was able to utilize my communication skills, drawing on the confidence that came so naturally to me to help other people in their cancer journeys. At last, long after my own cancer experience had been resolved, I'd found in cancer advocacy a real and meaningful way I could "fight" against cancer.

Advocacy helped me recognize that having cancer was far from a weakness, a liability or a waste of time as I had thought before. In fact, having cancer was a valuable set of skills and experiences which, when married with strengths and abilities I already had and others the Cancer Council helped develop, qualified me to do an important and effective work. By using my cancer experience as an asset and not a liability, I was able to help many others who must walk the same path as I had.

Whilst I personally didn't appreciate the "war on cancer" metaphor, I now understand how the imagery of the "cancer battle" can help many people better deal with cancer. It provides mental clarity and emotional inspiration, and also remakes cancer into something less intangible and abstract. One of the greatest dualities in cancer is the fact that the enemy is within you - the thing trying to kill you lies *inside your own body*. However, when you have cancer is exactly when your body needs your most delicate care and nurturing. Making cancer into an externalized and almost physically separate enemy with human attributes of personality and character gives many people something they can mount a campaign of resistance against, rather than their own bodies. Seeing cancer as a battle or a war can also help create a kind of distance between the person and the disease - *I am not this cancer.* In fact, I still take great care not to assign a cancer to a person by saying "his cancer, "her cancer" or "their cancer". We do not ask for, own or ever want the cancer. It comes of its own accord, we go to great pains to relieve ourselves of it, and we are all very glad to see the back of it. It is not "our cancer" – it is *the* cancer. This is one demonstration of how very simple words and ways of speaking can make a huge amount of difference to the way we think and behave.

I don't want to be brave any more.

When I changed the way I talked about cancer, it also changed my own expectations of myself. In thinking of cancer as more like a long, arduous journey I would one day reach the end of, I felt I didn't have to be as strong or brave as if I was fighting a war. I could allow myself to rest and recoup, or even to complain without feeling like I'd failed. Finding my own metaphor helped me explore my beliefs and feelings about having cancer, and also let me know *I couldn't do it wrong.* Being weak or emotional was not failing. When we are diagnosed, it can feel like the script for what we are allowed to say and do is already written for us, and lots of people make it their special job to remind us when we forget our lines. *Don't talk like that, you need to stay positive. What doesn't kill you makes you stronger. God has a reason for everything that happens to us.* These kinds of comments can suggest the person is failing if they don't see some overarching purpose in their illness, or if they aren't using it as an opportunity for self-improvement. Open conversations, rather than scripted promptings, help a person with cancer explore their genuine feelings about what's happening to them, and can also help them create their own mental analogy to describe their experience.

Why not write a cancer manifesto? The following is a suggested template for a cancer manifesto you may want to use as writing or a thinking exercise, and you could even us it as a mantra or an affirmation.

This is a (chapter, lap, round, path) in this cancer _____ (fight, journey, lesson, episode, war) etc.)

I thought cancer would be _____ (harder, tougher, weaker, easier, etc.)

Cancer has turned out to be _____ (crap, my teacher, a battle, a waste of time, etc.)

This is what cancer did –

This is what is will never do -

This is what it brought with it -

This is what it took away -

This is how I feel about it -

This will never be the same -

This will never change -

This is what I'll do now -

This is what will happen in the future –

This may prove to be a useful exercise in determining exactly what cancer means to you, and how you define and respond to it.

I'll conclude this chapter with a cancer manifesto by my friend John.

"Cancer is a rude, uninvited visitor. It didn't ask for my permission before it showed up, and when it did it made a nuisance of itself, so I won't make the mistake of thinking I must always show it my most perfect manners. I treat cancer with the same disdain and indifference I would any person whose company I can't stand. I'll laugh myself silly at its expense. I'll make it ashamed when I cry like a baby in front of it. I'll make it pay whenever the opportunity arises. I'll get as angry as I like and shout at it - with profanity if it makes me feel better. I refuse to empower it with my brave bearing up in its presence. I'll talk like it isn't here, because by all accounts one day it won't be, and by

gosh, I don't want it to have been the most exciting thing that ever happened to me when it finally does get out of town. And get out of town it will, because there's only room for one of us around here, and I'm not leaving anytime soon."

Bravo John, bravo. ☺

8

Things Not To Give To Someone Who Has Cancer.

I have a box in the cupboard I should probably think about throwing away soon. Not because it's full of junk like most of the boxes in the cupboard are, but because this particular box is way too small for its contents. Every time I take it out, I have to hold the lid in place and catch things as they fall out while I carry it across the room. Yep, I definitely need a bigger box for all those beautiful things people sent and gave to me when I had cancer back in 2003.

Cards. Notes. Letters. Drawings. A set of pictures sent home with one of my children from school created by their classmates, wishing me a quick recovery and telling me they were praying for me. I still become emotional looking at those drawings. A child's prayers are always as sincere and simple as their artwork, and I believe God is just as pleased with both these expressions.

Also in my box are little notes scribbled on scraps of paper I found pushed under my door, as well as store-bought, printed keepsakes sent to me by mail when I was hundreds of miles away from home. The memories these little tokens prompt are sometimes bittersweet. What a shame we often save the most honest expressions of our love until someone is ill. The feelings these objects evoke still surprise me with their intensity all these years later.

There are cards in that box from people whose faces I can't remember any more – customers from my shop and people I was acquainted with through church. I have letters in there from people who wrote how they had heard from friends of friends about what was happening to us and were praying, people I'd never met, and whom I never will. There is the book my thoughtful friend Wendy made for me, filled with lovely Victorian-style pictures and hand-written scriptures, and on whose empty pages I wrote my own answers to the many troubled questions I had. There is also a diary I tried so hard to keep with entries that stop around about the time my chemotherapy regime really kicked in. I remember feeling completely numb mentally and physically, and thinking I could never possibly want to read anything written during such a flat, featureless period of my life. It was as if the chemotherapy had not just interrupted the growth of all my physical cells but had somehow killed my creativity as well. Once a prolific songwriter, musician and artist, I felt *dry, dry, dry*. The abundance of others' creativity and generosity extended towards me buoyed me then, and still does today.

Over the months when I was having treatment, each time I would take out the box to add another card or note to it I would sit at the table and read every word others had written to me as if I were reading a beautiful story. In a time when I was numb and all my senses were blunted by loneliness and anxiety, reading those cards was like diving into clean, cold water. I'd forgotten what it felt like to *feel*, and those notes helped remind me again. Mattering enough to others for them to write it down gave me a reason to not simply lay down and shrivel up completely inside. Everything inside that box represents what was really important in my world.

Opening it up all these years later is like opening the window to a beautiful garden. It reminds me that I whilst ever I walk amongst the living, there is something worth living for. I think they call that *hope*.

*****

Being diagnosed with cancer can be an overwhelming experience – a kind of sensory and mental overload. Finding out you have cancer can answer some very pressing questions, but it can also bring with it more new information than you can possibly deal with all at once. Suddenly, life-altering decisions need to be made, each with possibly permanent consequences, and what you choose to do can turn out to be a matter of life and death. A cancer diagnosis can also herald the beginning of a sometimes intrusive and often painful treatment process. There may be times when the intensity of the experience is overwhelming, physically and emotionally, and other times when the monotony and repetition is mind numbing and incredibly frustrating. In between all the struggles a cancer patient has to make the right decisions and ask all the necessary questions, dealing with emotions and managing physical issues, there are other issues to think about as well. One of the most pressing ones is how your having cancer is affecting other people.

When you have cancer, *other people* are something you think about a lot. You think about not upsetting them, which ones you tell what to, about seeing some and not others and asking certain ones to do certain things for you. You think about getting them all together somehow, and getting them all to leave you alone. Other people often bring with their good intentions and generosity their own feelings about cancer, their opinions about what should be done about it, and perhaps even some pretty strong ideas about ways they're going to help. Sometimes they will help, a lot. But other times, the things people do can be a little bit confusing.

I was given some pretty random things when I had cancer, all of which were designed to help and make me feel better, but not all of them made it into my box. One lovely lady who I understood to be into New-Age spirituality came to the door with a few pictures of unicorns and other fantasy scenes she downloaded from the internet "for me to look at" - sweet, but baffling. Another dear friend gave me a massive jar of vitamin powder, and then there were those two identical copies of the very expensive cure-yourself-from-cancer diet book. It would have been rude for me to refuse such generous gifts outright. I felt obliged to accept them, even though I never used them.

When you bring your friend with cancer a present, they will

always appreciate it's done with the best of intentions. If the gift is unsuitable however, the recipient generally won't risk hurting your feelings by refusing your gesture. People may believe if they spend a lot of money on a gift, or if they believe it will help get rid of the cancer, it may be better received, but this isn't always the case. Here's a list of gifts, which, in my experience, you may want to think twice about.

Please do not give us a cancer-curing diet/meditation/affirmation book, particularly one we did not ask for.

These include books describing complex organic or raw food regimes, chanting certain affirmations or outlining daily prayer and meditation schedules. Whilst these diet and behavior modification plans may seem very practical and excellent to you, please consider that for most people a cancer diagnosis is a time of information overload. Our days may not be quite as empty as you think, and even if they are, we might not want to fill them with anything new. Also, however worried we may appear, providing us with more information will not necessarily solve our problems. As well, your choice of book will reflect your own values but may not reflect our own.

If you've heard about an alternative treatment, practice or theory by all means bring it up as a topic for an open discussion – and do this before you spent fifty dollars on the book and make a great gesture of presenting it to us. Allow the potential recipient of your gift the option to say "no thank you" or "yes, I'm interested" first.

Instate them as their own gatekeeper when it comes to the information they receive. Besides, with so many other people telling them what to do, it may well be that they'd really like you to be one of the ones who doesn't.

Please do not give us vitamin supplements, or alternative/herbal medications we did not specifically request.

There may be a very good reason we do not have these therapies in our medicine cabinet already. Many seemingly harmless and "natural" supplements and alternative treatments contain ingredients contra-indicated to mainstream medications prescribed to treat cancer. This means that even apparently innocuous tablets and tonics can work against prescribed treatments, and can even cause dangerous side effects such as blood clotting. Anyone under the care of a health professional must inform their practitioner if they plan to take vitamins or alternative therapies **before** they do so. It is unwise to offer your friend any additional therapies, supplements or medications without the patient having sought the advice of their health professional or clinician.

Please do not forward or print out that spam email.

If we could somehow get back all the wasted hours people have spent creating vexatious, inaccurate, over-sentimental and scare-mongering emails and social media status updates about cancer and channel them into something more positive I'm sure we'd have cured all the cancer in the known universe by now. These chain emails and cut-and-paste social media statuses can cause unnecessary worry, and are a very real emotional trigger for many people who have cancer or know someone with it. They can also contain wildly inaccurate information about cancer and its causes. Please don't forward them, no matter how pretty the animations or harrowing the stories.

Other things not to give to someone who has cancer.

- Heavily perfumed toiletry/bath products. Some people become highly sensitive to scented toiletries or those containing certain ingredients when they are having cancer treatments. Once my own chemotherapy started I found I couldn't stand certain smells I used to like. Before you buy, ask if there is anything they cannot tolerate or have developed an aversion to.

- Hats, wigs, headscarves or prosthetic items, unless specifically requested. This can be interpreted as overly familiar, or in bad taste.

- Books about people who either died tragically from or heroically survived cancer,[††] unless specifically requested. They may not be as "inspiring" as you think.

[††] One exception I would make to the "no cancer book" rule is Quest For Life, by Petrea King. Petrea is an Australian leukemia survivor and therapeutic practitioner offering both a holistic and realistic approach to living - and dying - with cancer. I recommend her book, but as with any book you plan to give, please do some homework first then introduce the idea of the book via an open conversation before offering to purchase it.

- Stories about your fabulous new job, your imminent holiday to Bali, your new house or your being promoted into their position at work because they had to take leave to have surgery and chemo. Great news is a subjective concept. Don't make this any harder than it needs to be.

- Anecdotes about new fake boobs, your facelift, the site of your last Botox or your liposuction scars. Stories about, and exhibitions of, unnecessary cosmetic surgical procedures can make a person who has endured a life-saving and necessary surgical procedure feel a little bit cranky.

- A Bible, or other books about positive thinking, spirituality or life after death. Unless they've asked you specifically asked you for them, they may think you're hastening them on to an afterlife.

- Sympathy cards. Yes, this really happens.

- A DVD copy of "Beaches", or any other film where someone tragically dies of cancer.

Things you can give to someone who has cancer.

- Chocolate. They can always share it with others if they can't have it.

- A nice bottle of wine - if they drink and are allowed alcohol. If they can't drink it, again, they can share it.

- Something in their size, just not a prosthetic bra, hat, wig or headscarf.

- A book about anything other than cancer. Perhaps something by their favorite author, or a book they've specifically asked you for.

- Cards, notes and letters with sincere good wishes. Don't get all maudlin and depressing, or make your correspondence into an opportunity to unburden yourself of all your sad feelings. Keep it light and heartfelt.

- Quilts - particularly the hand-made kind. My friends got together and made me a quilt, and I dragged that thing everywhere with me during treatment. I threw up on it, wrapped myself in it, showed it to everyone who would stand still long enough and then hung it up on the wall, where it remains to this day. A quilt can also be a wonderful gift for a friend whose outcome is not so promising. I gave a very ill friend of mine a quilt I made for him in his last few weeks of life. After he passed away, his wife had something lovely to take home from the hospital other than just his pyjamas and slippers.

- Blankets. Knee rugs. Pieces of beautiful fabric. Anything lovely you can keep warm inside and cuddle up to, or which you can make into something warm and cuddly, and can be machine-washed. I'm not personally a fan of soft toys, but go there if your friend likes them.

- A book of puzzles or word games, if they're the puzzle solving type. There's often a lot of waiting involved when you're having cancer treatment.

- A journal and a nice, operational pen. A brand new book of art paper and some pencils or pastels. A disposable camera. Anything that will help them record their journey or share their story in their own way.
- A book with messages from friends inside.
- A gift voucher for two for their local cinema.
- The kind of bathing and moisturizing products usually marketed to geriatrics or small babies, and not because they have pictures of roses or lavender on the labels. Ingredients are key. See first on the list of things not to buy.
- A hot, nutritious meal, delivered to the door, with a phone call first. Just check they haven't had four lasagna already that week.

Things to remember -

- *A good gift helps, not hinders.* If your gift is likely to add complexity to their lives instead of resolving it, think again. A quilt is good, but a gift certificate for a course of quilting classes over six consecutive Thursday evenings in the middle of winter on the other side of town is perhaps *not so much*. Give something that will solve problems, not create them.

- *If in any doubt, just ask first.* Your friend would probably rather be asked prior to your gift giving and forgo the surprise than have a less-than-happy surprise come their way.

- ***Keep it simple, keep it sincere.*** My shoe-box is filled with pieces of paper, cards and other inexpensive keepsakes, and they are treasures to me. The more they reminded me of the person who gave them to me, the more I wanted to keep them around. Someone I love an awful lot lent me a huge juicer, but I never used it and couldn't keep it so it had to go back, and the expensive diet books were sold on EBay. Grand or expensive gestures do not always have the impact you imagine they will.

- ***Their values, not yours.*** If you are of the same faith persuasion or religion, then a book of scriptures or by an author you both enjoy is probably appropriate. If they are vegan, a vegetable steamer is also suitable. However, anything you give them, which subtly suggests your faith/diet/religion/exercise regime is superior to theirs and would in your opinion improve their likelihood of surviving cancer, is probably closer to propaganda, and unsuitable.

- ***All they really want is you.*** Your friend or loved one will most likely be very contented simply to spend quality time with you whenever they are able. You don't need to feel obligated to give them presents, because it may not be anything you can wrap in paper they are craving right now. Sometimes a few moments of honest silence, or just sitting together without questions or expectations, is the most precious thing you can offer. In fact, the best thing you can give to someone who has cancer is not actually a thing – it's *you.* ☺

9

"You've changed."
Why people who have cancer
don't always go back to normal.

When a person is diagnosed with cancer, everyone believes there are only two possible outcomes. The first one we don't even want to think about – it's the outcome everyone wants to avoid - *dying of cancer*. The other outcome is the one everyone wants – *for cancer to go away and everything to just go back to normal*. Most people assume that if outcome number one doesn't happen, then outcome two will just naturally come about. So cancer treatment is finished and the crisis is over. Doesn't everything just go back to the way it was before?

Everyone diagnosed with cancer hopes one day they will not just be well from cancer, but also perhaps hopes their life can be just like it was before ever cancer came along. We might even think this is the way we'll know it's finally all over – when everything returns to "normal". But sometimes things don't go back to normal. Sometimes things are never the same again, and one of those things can be the person who had cancer.

When they told me I was no longer likely to die from lymphoma, I knew exactly what I wanted – to get back home from treatment to my family, my church and my job as soon as possible. The "cancer world" was not a place I planned to spend any more time than I absolutely had to, thank you very much. When someone suggested it might help me if I found a cancer support group, I told them emphatically *no thanks*. Sitting around with a bunch of people complaining about cancer was the last thing I wanted to do. The world of treatment, hospitals and other people with cancer was not somewhere I wanted to stay, and I certainly didn't want to make any friends there. As far as I was concerned, when my treatment was finished, everything was to return to the way it was before, and it would be like cancer had never happened.

Many years later, having spent quite some time after I went into remission in counseling for depression and anxiety, as well as a few years volunteering extensively in the cancer sphere, I realized that despite never wanting to stay in the "cancer world" I had in fact never left it. I never did go back to "normal", but completely reinvented my life from top to bottom. Despite what I'd hoped would occur, because of and even thanks to cancer, my life had completely changed, and would never be the same again.

There were many reasons I found I could not simply return to the way things used to be. Everything was different, including me. I had new information about the world and the kinds of things that can happen to people. I'd experienced some things many people never experience. I'd been more afraid and more in pain than ever before in my life, and I'd seen people I'd grown to care for deeply suffer and sometimes die. I'd plumbed my own spiritual and emotional depths, and seen the very best and worst in others as well. My priorities had changed. I didn't want the same things I had before. By the time I finished my treatment, what once was important to me no longer mattered, and I found myself desperately wanting to do things I'd never given myself permission to try. My life was in flux. I realized there was no "going back to normal". I had to find a *new normal.*

*****

Quite early on after someone is diagnosed with cancer we may begin to talk about the idea of everything returning to "normal". As I mentioned at the beginning of this chapter, this is probably because in everyone's mind the alternative doesn't bear thinking about. But for the person with cancer, and even for the people who love them, it may not be as simple as just picking up exactly where they left off before the diagnosis. Cancer can affect a person in subtle ways, and the mental and emotional scars can be as painful and lasting as any of the physical ones.

Sometimes, people around the person with cancer can apply subtle pressure to "get over it" as quickly as possible, but it may not be as simple as everyone hopes or expects. A cancer experience can change a person in very deep and fundamental ways, and the pressure of being expected to forget everything that happened on the journey can be hard to deal with. Any changes perhaps cannot be simply reversed or ignored, but may need to be recognized, acknowledged and managed supportively.

There is also a common expectation that if cancer changes a person it is always for the better. Many people assume a cancer experience facilitates a personal transformation experience, and thus we emerge from cancer more evolved, understanding and at peace with ourselves and everyone else around us. It's also generally assumed we are all able to make some kind of sense of our cancer experience, and enjoy nothing better than sharing the moral of our cancer story for the benefit of everyone else. Church people sometimes like to call this a "testimony". Despite these myths, sometimes people do not become better for having had cancer. In fact, I've found the positive personal transformation is totally optional.

Cancer can be the making of a person, but it can also be the breaking of them.

Some folks become extremely self-focused during and after their cancer experience, and while this often settles down over time, what sometimes results is a permanent reorganization of priorities. Spouses, families and careers may be abandoned, and lives that were ordered and organized beforehand may be wrecked, even deliberately. This is very difficult to witness, let alone be subjected to. When massive changes follow a cancer experience, it can come as a surprise. However, the kinds of issues bringing about such changes are usually underlying the whole time, and cancer is often merely the catalyst or an opportunity for change.

As both a cancer patient and a cancer support program facilitator, I have come to appreciate how varied different peoples' cancer journeys can be. Whilst some people seem to sail through their cancer experience without any significant problems, others are so traumatized by it they need to seek counseling and support. I was one of the latter. Several months after my treatment was over, when everything "should" have been back to normal, I found myself caught in a whirlpool of anxiety and indecision. I catastrophized about minor decisions and was unable to move forward. For example, my husband Ben was desperate to take our family away on a camping holiday, but I just couldn't commit. I was absolutely terrified of being any distance away from my doctor, and I couldn't imagine how a rescue helicopter would land at the camping ground if something terrible happened to me. Of course, these thoughts were quite irrational, but for me they were absolutely justifiable. In counseling, I was able to recognize my anxiety was significantly affecting my ability to make simple choices. We worked to increase my confidence to the point where I was able to go on holidays with my family again, and we even moved to the next town, where I would need to travel an hour to visit my doctor. This for me was a major step forward.

Several years after I sought counseling for my post-treatment anxiety, I began facilitating a Cancer Council program called Living Well After Cancer[‡‡], designed to help cancer survivors[§§]

[‡‡] The Living Well After Cancer Program is a free community education program, developed by Cancer Council NSW (Australia) and delivered by fully trained cancer survivors. Information can be found on the Cancer Council website at www.cancercouncil.com.au

orientate themselves within their journey. LWAC supports survivors to make strategies for moving forward into their "new normal". An important part of the program is providing ways for people to debrief about what's happened to them. Participants often share how family and friends enthusiastically encourage them to "get on with their life" and not talk about the past. This is often because past cancer experiences are very painful for family and friends to hear about, and can trigger strong emotions. If a cancer patient or survivor feels they need to talk about their experiences, it's important they find an avenue for this. It may be they have some supportive friends and family who are able to provide a listening ear, but if not, they may need to discuss this with their doctor or seek out a qualified counselor.

Sometimes it isn't the person with the cancer who struggles to get back to normal - it's the carer, spouse or loved one. Almost two years after my cancer went into remission, my husband Ben went to see our doctor with feelings of depression and general emotional flatness for which he was prescribed anti-depressants. It was another two years before it became apparent to all of us that Ben had become an alcoholic, and by then our marriage had practically fallen apart. The cancer was long gone and I was well again, but

---

§§ "Survivor" is a term I commonly use to describe people in the treatment or post-treatment phase of cancer, but not everyone who has experienced cancer likes to be known as such. "Survivors" will usually self-identify as such, but in a support group or clinical context it is not advised to use this word to generally describe all persons who have had/currently have cancer without first gaining a consensus.

now it was Ben's turn to plunge into personal crisis. He was admitted into a residential rehab program, and whilst there was able to identify how my having cancer triggered feelings of inadequacy and despair in him he simply lacked the resources to deal with. With support, we've since been able to put our marriage back together and move forward. Ben's journey through cancer was just as impacting as mine, despite the fact it wasn't him with the diagnosis. After eight years, we have not returned to any semblance of our lives before I was sick. We've had to recreate our marriage and our family life with all the new information we have about ourselves and about the world. We're stronger now, and wiser, but also more wary. Never again will I take my husbands strength for granted, nor my own health or happiness.

Few can walk a tough path like cancer and not be changed somehow, and it's hard when others don't welcome the changes cancer can bring. Locating a supportive and symbiotic cancer community with whom we can share our experiences is another reason to find a good support group. Despite my initial misgivings, I found talking to other cancer survivors was like finding lost members of a tribe. We shared similar memories. We spoke the same language. We didn't have to interpret medical terms or explain diagnoses to each other. Often we'd find we knew the same people and had been to the same places. Connecting about common cancer ground helped normalize my experiences and reassured me that I wasn't weird or broken for thinking and feeling a certain way. Contrary to what I'd believed, not a lot of whining goes on at cancer support groups. There is however an awful lot of laughing.

It's hard to imagine travelling overseas on a long trip or taking a job across the country and not being allowed to talk about it when you come back, but for many people who have cancer, this is exactly what happens. Friends and family often do not welcome conversations about cancer, and may fear the person is "dwelling on the past" or not "moving on". Counseling and support groups can be a way for people to talk about their cancer experience with those who understand and share their experiences, without appearing to be holding onto the past or making cancer into their permanent identity. As well, the memories of the cancer may be interesting and positive for the patient, but may be very painful or aggravating for the carer. I had a lady who came along religiously to our support group every month, but whose husband stayed in the car and read the paper the whole time. It was her chance to talk about her feelings and her illness openly without causing her husband any undue anxiety. Both were very happy with the arrangement.

In starting my own cancer support group, I discovered it isn't just sick and old people who join these groups. All kinds of people came to ours - carers, partners, support people, best friends, sons, daughters, siblings and parents. Support groups fulfill many different functions for their members. Some are social gatherings, whilst some can be more intense, and rather like group counseling sessions. Others can be exclusive and closed like private clubs. Some groups use their time together and their talents to become involved in fundraising and cancer charity work. Many of those who attend support groups find them to be a way they can stay in the "cancer world" and keep the friends they made there whilst transitioning into the next phase of their journey. Whilst the idea of support groups may not hold appeal for many patients and survivors, it's important to realize that a cancer experience is always significant one, and support can comes in many different forms.

- *For cancer patients/survivors* – If you feel you'd like to talk about aspects of your cancer experience with someone and you don't feel your family and friends are the appropriate avenue, please consult with your doctor or health professional about counseling or support services in your locale. You could also check with a social worker at your hospital, or with a cancer support charity or agency to see what may be available for your specific cancer type or phase of treatment.

- *For family members, carers, partners and other support persons* – Carers and family members closely involved with a person who has cancer can be deeply impacted by the experience as well. As a carer, you will need not just emotional support, but may even require practical support as well. Cancer can be extremely physically draining and anxiety producing, and carers need to take care of their own well-being. Many cancer support groups are not just for the person with cancer, and most allow carers, friends and supporters to come along, even on their own. Please check with your local support group to see if they cater for carers. There are also support groups in some areas specifically for carers and family members, and some which cater for carers and partners of those who are palliative. In our town, we even have a grieving partners support group. To find such a group, please check in the phone book, with a social worker connected with your hospital, or contact your doctor. Look around your doctors' waiting room for flyers. You may also find some support services for carers directly through cancer charities and support services.

While we all want cancer to go away with as few reminders and consequences as possible, this does not always happen. Cancer can leave physical as well as emotional scars, and these must be acknowledged and supported wherever and however they occur. Sometimes the "old normal" of the pre-cancer life is gone forever, and a "new normal" needs to be found to replace it. While the impact of decisions made in the wake of cancer can be drastic and permanent, those changes do not always have to be negative, and denial can be just as damaging as self-sabotage. It's important for those recovering from cancer as well as their supporters and family to seek appropriate counseling where necessary, and acknowledge the individual processes taken to move through the experience with universal compassion and understanding.

Things to remember –

- *Some folks never go back to normal after cancer - the best they can do is to find a new normal.*

- *When someone has cancer, they don't always become a "better" person as a result. They may be changed emotionally, physically or psychologically in any number of ways, and can also become more anxious or depressed as they leave the relative security of treatment and follow-up appointments.*

- *Many of the psycho-social issues which arise during cancer and treatment can exacerbate pre-existing psychological problems or addictions. Both the diagnosed person and their carers need to be careful to maintain their support systems, and seek help where required from trained health and counseling services.*

- *It isn't always the person with the cancer who struggles to find the new normal. It can be the carer, partner family member and even the children who need support to transition to the post-cancer phase of the disease.*

- *A social worker, your doctor, a counseling provider or cancer support service may refer you or suggest support groups and/or counseling programs suitable for the post-treatment phase of the disease, for both patients and carers.* ☺

10

Things Never To Say To Someone Who Has Cancer
God, spirituality, death
and other tangled balls of existential string.

Up to this point, we've discussed things not to say to someone who has cancer in terms of general clichés and false premises. We've examined ways of initiating conversations about cancer, demystifying and diffusing the fear and anxiety surrounding it, and finding practical ways to help our friend or loved one through the use of open questions. We've unpacked some of the language people use when discussing cancer, and also considered some new ways of talking and thinking about it. We've also examined some of the reasons why the people we love who have cancer sometimes behave contrary to our expectations. After visiting a few of these peripheral topics, it's time to revisit the original theme of this book. Before the final chapter, we'll now drill down into the Things Not To Say To Someone Who Has Cancer a little deeper, and discuss the subject from a slightly different angle.

Whilst some of the specific things I've already identified as Things Not To Say are not particularly logical, they aren't especially offensive. This would include things like –

"You need to stay positive."

"What doesn't kill you makes you stronger."

"My cousin had that, and they died."

From a person with cancers' point of view, these phrases may be annoying, but are unlikely to cause deep distress or offence and were obviously never intended to. There are however a particular type of phrase or cancer clichés to avoid saying to your friend or loved one who has cancer, because the possible offense and distress caused may be far more significant. The first type I'll describe includes statements along the following lines –

"God/The Universe is teaching you something."

"Cancer is caused by stress/sin/unforgiveness/toxic thoughts/emotions."

"Cancer never happens to people who *<insert religious practice here>*."

"God wants to use this for His glory."

"If you pray and have enough faith, God will heal you."

"God will never give us more than we can handle."

Let's address this particular type of cliché first.

It's my experience that this type of platitude seldom helps in the way the person intended, and unlike the lesser cliché's which are far more benign, may actually cause considerable upset, confusion and distress.

Now, before we go any further, I'd like to explain this chapter is in no way intended to be accusatory or condemning. I'm not trying to make the family and friends of someone with cancer feel ashamed, inadequate, judged or guilty. Both I, and the people these things are said to every single day, appreciate that when it happens it's without any intention to hurt or harm. In fact, as in the case of most cancer clichés, the things are frequently spoken simply because the person doesn't know what else to say. However, the carelessness with which they are used can belie the upset they can potentially cause.

When something tragic, unexpected or terrible frightens us a little bit more than usual, its common for us to start thinking about the deeper meaning of life. Fear of feeling out of control can have us turning our thoughts to spiritual things. However, as with more tangible matters, clichés are quite inadequate to articulate or initiate conversations about such things. As we've already discussed, clichés generally contain elements of truth, but in and of themselves they are not *the* truth. Further, clichés act in a conversation to close a subject down. When you're on a personal or spiritual quest for answers, you're looking for open doors, and not brick walls. This is why clichés are generally useless in addressing significant issues such as cancer, and are particularly redundant in this context.

There is another more malignant aspect of the pseudo spiritual cancer cliché. Whilst most clichés can be shrugged off as impersonal or simply not applicable, the particular examples given above may subtly infer the person caused their own cancer through something they did or did not do – specifically, something spiritual, emotional or relational in nature. The overarching implication is if the person had thought, felt or behaved contrary to the way they did, they would not have become ill in the first place. They also suggest reversing or changing the behavior concerned, replacing it with a different behavior or practice or at least acknowledging behavior or attitudes are responsible, will get rid of the cancer. This is a wholly subjective – and even dangerous – concept, and hopefully it's quite clear why it is inappropriate to imply someone caused their own cancer, inadvertently or otherwise. In a nutshell, *it hurts to be told cancer is your own fault.* Statements along these lines are disempowering, not encouraging or supportive, and only cause shame and guilt. Further, every person has the right to come to their own conclusions about their having cancer, and decide for themselves what meaning, if any, the experience has for them.

Most people I know who have cancer spend at least some time wondering if they caused it through something they did or didn't do, particularly if there is no physical explanation or obvious cause. *What did I do to make this happen? Did I take a wrong turn somewhere? Am living outside of Gods will? Did I cause this because I refused to forgive that person who hurt me? Am I in a bad relationship? What does this mean? Is this my fault?* The kinds of folks with thoughts like these seldom need someone else to point these issues out to them – they can do it all on their own. They certainly don't need anyone weighing in with more. What they require is support from a non-judgmental source, an opportunity to discuss their thoughts and feelings and come to their own conclusions. I also know many people with cancer who don't give these kinds of thoughts any weight at all. For them, cancer is a purely physical and not a psychic disorder. In either situation a pseudo spiritual cliché is of no use whatsoever.

While many of us profess some kind of spirituality, we will all express – and must be permitted to express - our spirituality in different ways. Many people use theology and religion as a way to understand the world around them, and provide an explanation for the confusing things in life. When it comes to my own personal faith expression, as a Christian I believe in God, but I realize not everyone shares my beliefs. My own exploration and personal understanding of my illness has been helpful for me, however my interpretations have not turned out to be transferable to others. The conclusions I've come to about my own having cancer came many years later after much reflection on the disease, my treatment and the years following afterwards. I found I had little perspective on the spiritual or psychological implications of my having cancer whilst I was living it, and the meaning I have been able to draw from has taken almost a decade for me to clarify.

Trudy works for a cancer charity, and is eight years out from her own cancer experience. The breast cancer spread down her arm past her wrist, and resulted in disfiguring surgery. Trudy's strong personality and cheeky sense of humor is perfect for her job in health promotion, and when she's around there is always lots of laughter. While Trudy has no problem encouraging others to not take cancer too seriously, I found when it comes to discussing her own experience, she becomes withdrawn and reflective. "I know why I got cancer," she tells me, "I was very harsh on my son when he was a teenager, and I was always on his back about stupid little things. Our relationship was almost ruined when I found out I had breast cancer. I believe it was my critical attitude that caused the disease, and I've had to work hard both to get well again, and to repair my relationship with my boy." For her, Trudy's cancer experience was a wake-up call for her regarding her priorities, and showed her what is really important in her life. In telling me her story, Trudy wasn't seeking my affirmation about what caused the cancer – she has already identified what for her was the cause, and has actively set herself work to do. Trudy's relationship with her son is now greatly improved as a result, and she believes the cancer had no reason to come back.

When I had cancer, I went along to church just as I normally did. Despite the fact not many of my fellow church-goers knew me intimately, I found people often remarked in conversation that they believed cancer was an attempt by God to teach me a lesson, make me stronger, have me be a "witness" to others or provide me with an interesting testimony, amongst other things. After saying these things, the people who said them promptly went away and completely forgot about it, leaving me to consider the weight of their statement and its implications for me. It took me a long time to realize they didn't really believe what they'd said to me, it was simply something to say – something which didn't sound as glib or trivial as other things they might have said, and which seemed meaningful and conveyed their deep concern. However, whenever someone said to me "God is trying to teach you something" it felt kind of like being told I was now enrolled in a class with no subject, no classroom and no teacher, and my grades had better be good – or else. *What am I supposed to be learning? How will I know if I've graduated? What happens if I fail the exam?*

After I was well again, people invited me to speak to their church groups about my *testimony*, but I didn't feel I had really one. I had no idea why I had cancer, and I still didn't know what lesson – if any – God had been trying to teach me through it. Also, I didn't think I was a stronger or better person because I'd had cancer – I'd left my successful career and was now unemployed, my husband was on anti-depressants and I was riddled with anxieties about the cancer coming back. Besides, how could I claim God had healed me when I'd had chemotherapy and radiotherapy? After a while, I avoided talking to spiritual-minded people about having cancer, because I always felt as though they expected me to give it a deeper meaning, and I didn't have one. Worse, many of them wanted to endow the cancer I had with some deep meaning of their own, usually made up on the spot without any insight into my life or my own personal beliefs.

Faith in God and other kinds of spiritual practice can help people make sense of a cancer experience. Many find comfort in their faith when they are going through cancer and treatment, but many will be challenged and perhaps even discard former practices. I've heard from several families whose children were ill with cancer on how the experience sorely tested their beliefs. Some conclude that a God who allows children to suffer and die is not worthy of their worship, whilst others will press in and draw more deeply on their faith for courage and meaning. Neither of these approaches can be judged as better than the other, but as loved ones and supporters we can offer to lend our strength and compassion in whatever capacity we feel is called for. Glib, faux-spiritual comments and simplistic clichés certainly have no place in situations like these.

In fact, I struggle to think of any situation where they do have a place.

Having said all of this, the true irony of the pseudo spiritual cliché is that while they may sound like the most meaningful thing to say, they are most often said without any real conviction - religious, moral or otherwise. These phrases are loaded with subtle connotations which are usually the exact opposite of what the person saying them intends to communicate. In most cases the person doesn't truly believe God is trying to teach us something, or that our thoughts and emotions caused the cancer – what they really mean is "I don't know why this happened, but I do know it's important, and it matters a lot. I need to convey the seriousness of how I feel about this to you the only way I know how." People are terrified of saying something trite and meaningless, so instead they say something they hope will reflect the depth and gravity of how they feel. God and cancer can both make people feel terrified and out of control, and I think this is one reason they so frequently end up in the same sentence.

Evangelizing or "witnessing" to someone who has cancer.

A cancer experience can be a time of deep reflection and change for everyone concerned. Our faith both in God and in other people, and even in ourselves, can be deeply challenged. We may require spiritual or emotional guidance and support to help us through this time, and we may trust the people around us to help us access or provide that support. Whilst most efforts to bring spiritual meaning to a cancer experience are simply attempts to comfort the person with the cancer, many see a vulnerable person as an opportunity to introduce their own particular religious or spiritual perspectives. Whilst evangelizing or "witnessing" to someone with cancer may come from pure motives, we must be very, very careful of using someone's cancer experience as a point of entry for a religious conversion.

I am aware that a good many people, many of whom share my particular faith expression, will disagree with me on this point. I recognize many folks feel they have a moral obligation to their friend or loved one with cancer to provide spiritual perspectives and guidance particularly if the person involved is reaching the end of their life. Sharing on matters of spirituality and encouraging one another in our faith is certainly a healthy part of human relations, however we must also remember that subtlety, respect and acceptance are equally important. In all matters of faith and spirituality, when it comes to your loved one with cancer please, *tread lightly.*

When I say it's unwise to bring up spiritual matters with a cancer patient, I am not talking about the general admonitions of professional ministers, counselors or chaplains. Qualified people in appointed positions will be clearly identified as such, and may not approach a patient unless invited to do so. If their pastoral assistance or guidance is not required, a patient is well within social and personal parameters to decline. A healthy pastoral relationship is one where permission is sought to discuss certain matters, qualified responses and guidance are offered and not imposed, and the person receiving the ministry guides the discussion with their own needs and questions.

"My friend wants to talk about the spiritual implications of having cancer. What do I say?"

For me, the key to discussing matters of spirituality with a person who has cancer is to compassionately support their search for answers, without forcing or questioning their methods or their conclusions. It's okay to ask questions of God, to want to know why, to be angry sometimes and feel as if life has treated us unjustly, and this doesn't mean we have abandoned God, or have no faith. When someone we love has deeper questions, rather than feeling we need to provide clear-cut answers, theological or otherwise, we can help by simply being present with them in amongst the confusion and hurt. There is much to be said for providing a non-judgmental ear to listen, and a compassionate hand to hold.

Other strategies for spiritual or holistic support -

- Remember your open questions, and avoid making closed statements. If your friend indicates they'd like to talk about the more spiritual aspects of their cancer journey, rather than saying, "I think _____", or presenting your own interpretation of their experience, ask them "What do you think?" Don't be intimidated by feeling you need to provide answers. Perhaps a resolution will come in time. Cancer is not a test or exam they can fail.

- In asking questions of this kind, they may be sending you a signal about the way they are really feeling emotionally or physically. People often draw on their faith in times of deep anxiety and fear. Think about ways you may be able to allay their fear or soothe their anxiety with reassuring words and comforting actions. Hugs are good.

- If they wish to talk about the spiritual implications of their experiences, provide ways for them to unpack their own thoughts and feelings, rather than offering statements that attempt to explain everything away. Allow them to articulate their fear or anger, rather than requiring they hold it in or hide it. They may be afraid of disappointing or frightening you. Giving them permission to express the full scope of their emotions can create an atmosphere of security and acceptance.

- Encourage them to undertake activities designed to relax them physically and mentally, and help them to feel nurtured and settled. Sometimes the only physical experiences a cancer patient has are painful ones. Where suitable, a massage, yoga, a warm bath or a meditation session may help them feel more comfortable and soothed.

- Invite them on a spiritual excursion. Offer to take them somewhere they have a positive spiritual or emotional connection to, or where they feel relaxed and happy. Sitting at a lookout, watching the ocean, visiting a church or connecting with other people may help them feel more settled and safe.

Now, let's move on to the second kind of cliché never to say. This other category includes the following clichés, or things sounding like them -

"Everyone has to die of something."

"Well, at least they're in a better place now."

Cancer inevitably makes our thoughts turn to death and dying. When it comes to cancer, death is always a possibility. More and more people are surviving cancer, but the worst possible case scenario still haunts us all. Despite all the advances in treatment, the truth remains that for many people diagnosed with cancer, the disease will result in their physical demise.

In other words, some people diagnosed will die of cancer.

If we were not afraid of dying and death, cancer wouldn't inspire such dread in us. Of course we're afraid. We're afraid of the pain, the loss and the deep unknown that may or may not lie beyond it. If we weren't afraid cancer might kill us, we wouldn't need to talk about it in language usually reserved for military conflict, and we wouldn't need to be so scared about saying the wrong things to people when they have it.

Dying is the great fear every person diagnosed with cancer harbors, secretly or not so secretly. A person with cancer must confront the possibility of their own death at some stage, even if it's just to decide where they stand in relation to it. We might reasonably expect that everyone diagnosed with cancer wants to avoid death, at least at first. For many, the time comes when the inevitability of death is no longer abstract and distant, but is something we must prepare ourselves for as an approaching reality.

In Western society, for the most part, we have no idea how to talk about death. We pussyfoot around it with our words and our euphemisms, and go to great lengths to put it off even when our bodies have lost the capacity to sustain life without medical intervention. Death is coming to all of us, however one of the things not to say to someone who has cancer is "Oh well, we all have to die of something". This is not so much a matter of avoidance as it is of respect. Death absolutely must be talked about, but those who have lived knowing death is coming, or have lived amongst the dying, know not to talk of death so lightly.

Everyone has probably remarked at some time or another *"Oh, but we're all dying"*, but we don't really mean what we say. The irony contained in this statement hinges on it being uttered by someone who will go to bed tonight, get up tomorrow morning and look out with optimism on a life they could reasonably expect to span at least a few more productive years. *We're all dying, but I still have time for living.* A person with cancer may not feel they have the luxury of speaking so flippantly about death under the circumstances, and it behooves us to extend to them the courtesy of not speaking this way in their presence.

I find these days I cannot say with any conviction *we're all dying*. I have known people who were dying, and what they were doing was nothing like what I do every day. Being with people who were consciously dying changed my whole perspective on my cancer experience, and on my own life and death. When I saw what it looks and feels like to be dying, I developed a new appreciation for what it means to be fully alive. From that time onwards, I knew I always wanted to do it – be fully alive that is - at least for as long as I possibly could.

The most impacting eight weeks in my life was the time I spent living in a hostel in Sydney with a group of people undergoing radiotherapy at the same time as me. When I arrived, I assumed everyone was doing what I was doing – going through the motions of treatment, and hopefully going home again at the end of it with both the cancer and the treatment finished with forever. But after a few weeks it became clear whilst some of us would be going home to pick up our lives where we left off, some of us would not. Some came expecting to go home after six weeks, but instead, came to a place of realizing this was the beginning of a new part of their life – the final part.

One morning, I went out to our shared kitchen for breakfast and was told the friendly little lady having treatment for mouth cancer would now be taking all her meals in her room from now on, assisted by her husband. *What changed?* The chatty middle-aged man who once waited with me at the bus stop suddenly started taking a taxi to the hospital by himself. *Why doesn't he want to talk to us any more?* The young woman who bragged about finishing these two months of treatment and just getting back to her friends and her job was now leaving after just four weeks, her bags packed and piled up outside her door. *Why isn't she finishing the radiotherapy?* We all arrived thinking this was just a phase we had to endure to go back our normal lives, but for some of us, there wasn't any going back to normal. This was the beginning of the end. Some of us went home to begin plans for a life beyond cancer. Some of us went home to make wills and get our affairs in order.

When I went home to my house filled with the warm, shouting, squirming bodies of my children, and I stood beside a new bed my wonderful husband made as a gift for me while I was away, I felt a sense of gratitude I'd never felt before. I was home, and I was alive. This would all go on, and I would be here to see it. I had been as close as all those others to death, but I'd come back and would now keep going. It was not the end for me - it was a new beginning. I would never again so glibly consider this wonderful existence – this second chance – to be anything resembling *dying*.

No, we are not all dying, but we are not all living either. What I saw in my friends at the hostel was the acceptance that there would be no new things any more, only the ending of things that were already begun. They began to withdraw from the world in small increments, newest things first. The friendships we formed in that time were those newest things, and probably the last things they would ever begin in their lives. When we said goodbye, we knew it was for the last time.

Those two months, and the years I've spent working with people who have cancer and seeing many of my close friends pass away, have all helped me confront my own fear of dying. I find I am far more afraid of wasting my life than I am of leaving it. However, seeing death so close-up, dreaming of it, smelling and hearing it all around me and then becoming so familiar as to recognize it in others has given me something in place of the fear. Respect. I deeply respect death, and it's because of this I cannot speak of it frivolously. It also alarms me when others presume to do so, particularly when they are speaking to someone for whom the proximity of death is a very real concern.

The other way we can trivialize death is by minimizing the impact it has on the ones who are left behind. My friend Sally recently related to me how, after her mother died of cancer, people commented to her "We should all feel better knowing she's in a better place now." Sally was appalled. Yes, her mother had a terrible time, and it was good to know she was not suffering any longer. But my friend had *lost her mother*, who had died far too young and in pain. Sally's loss and grief was real, and she needed comforting and a place to air the sense of injustice she felt about it. Sally, who believes in God and in Heaven, asked me "What is this *better place* my mother is in? What better place could there be than here with me?" The remarks Sally's friends made were intended only to help, but feeling she had no place to air her grief, she slumped deeper into depression. Sally felt deep sadness at her mothers passing, but she also felt ashamed for being angry about it. It only took a small prompting from me for Sally to pour out her emotions, relieved at last for permission to express her true thoughts and feelings without being placated or silenced.

However difficult we may find it to talk about death, the best way to deal with those difficulties is actually to talk about it some more. Whether a person has cancer, or is a carer or family member, we need to be mindful to give them permission with our words and actions to express their fears, anxieties and apprehensions without dismissing them as morbid or negative. Death is segmented off from many of us to the extent we can often go through life without ever seeing death first hand if we so choose. As a result, the mystique and fear surrounding death and the wide perception all death is bad or violent is rife. Not all death is bad, although some certainly is. It is possible to have a good death, and this will mean different things to different people.

Another issue we must be mindful of is the language we use in describing people who have died of cancer, as in when we say, "they lost their battle with cancer." In describing death in this way, dying becomes synonymous with giving in, with failure, weakness or a lack of will. Dying of cancer can be a kind of surrender, but it doesn't necessarily mean an adversary was victorious over us. More tragic than a person dying of cancer is speaking about the cancer as if between the two of them, cancer was the greater, or the stronger. Cancer may be the means by which we die, but may it never claim to be more formidable than we were in life. Cancer will never surpass us, and one day, perhaps even in our lifetime, will not exist at all. We may only hope.

Things to remember –

- *Most cancer cliché's are benign, and may cause little more than annoyance. However, the kind of cliché that glibly makes reference to more deeply personal issues such as spirituality, God, death and dying, should be avoided.*

- *Where concepts of intangible causes of the cancer such as emotional or spiritual are concerned, it's important to allow the person experiencing the disease to embark upon their own search for answers, and to lead that quest according to their own beliefs.*

- *Our role as a carer or supporter is to support the person in their own choices, and to act as a sounding board as they air their thoughts and feelings. While we are free and ought to contribute, in the end, it doesn't matter what we think about their cancer experience, why it happened, or what will happen because of it. It really only matters what they think about it.*

- *Whilst losing someone to cancer is always a terrible loss for family and friends, dying of cancer itself doesn't mean we have "lost" or failed. We can honor a person who has died of cancer by celebrating their lives, cherishing who they were and commemorating what they achieved, and also by fulfilling their wishes concerning the way they would like to be remembered. One way we can all work to reduce the fear that surrounds cancer is to find other ways of talking about it, including the way we talk about someone who dies from it. Death is certainly a kind of surrender, but dying of cancer does not necessarily mean we were defeated.*

- *Death is difficult to talk about and nobody likes being faced with the demise of someone they love, however it may be necessary at some time for you to discuss the spiritual, social and medical aspects of death and dying. These conversations may surround the planning of palliative care, services to be held after their passing or may be about more spiritual matters. If you feel out of your depth, seek support both for yourself, and for your loved one. Social workers, pastoral carers, chaplains, counselors and other support services are available through hospitals, support groups and cancer organizations.* ☺

11

The Conversation Continues.

This is the last chapter of the book I've wanted to write for so long about the Things Not To Say To Someone Who Has Cancer. To be honest with you, I haven't really been looking forward to writing this chapter. The last few words of any book can often seem like the "final word" on the subject. This may be exactly what the author intends, but I didn't write this book so I could have the final word about the things not to say to someone who has cancer. I also didn't write it to establish myself as the authority on the subject, or because I decided my opinions on the matter are the only ones that count. I wrote this book because I really want to help people – people with cancer, and the folks who love them. I wrote it because I've been in both sets of those shoes, and I understand just how confronting and confusing it can be. I wrote this book because I've felt for a long time it was something I could've really used myself along the way, whether as a cancer patient, or as a friend of someone who was diagnosed.

I hope it's clear by now I didn't write this book to mock those who may have said some of the things not to say I've highlighted, or to criticize helpers and carers. I've said every single one of the things not to say I've mentioned in this book, and plenty more besides, so I'm certainly not taking the higher ground. I've had all the things not to say said back to me as well, by people I loved and cared about, folks I just didn't have the heart to tell, "what you just said doesn't help as much as you probably hope, but I know what you meant". I wrote this book because again and again I've seen fear, apprehension and desperation on the face of someone who pulled me aside to ask me, "Please help me - my friend has just been diagnosed with cancer, and I have no idea what to say." I wrote this book because of the countless people I've heard express their sadness and confusion about their relationships, damaged sometimes beyond repair, after cancer came along. I wrote this book because so many people struggle with how to act or what to say when someone is diagnosed with cancer, and far too often we decide it's all just too hard. I wrote this book because I believe there are far better ways we can talk about cancer, and ways we can talk to people who have cancer than many of the ways we've tried in the past. Lots of the ways we've become very accustomed to using are not working, and I think we can do better.

So why is it better to talk about cancer, and to people who have cancer, in certain ways, but not in others? *Because we all want to help, and some of the old ways we talk about cancer don't help.* In fact, some of the old ways we talk about cancer *hurt.* They hurt emotionally, socially and relationally. They can give the impression people don't care, or don't care enough. They perpetuate old myths about cancer, and reinforce untruths and half-truths. They build walls where we need bridges, and create obstacles where we need pathways. An awful lot of the things we've said to people who had cancer in the past did the exact opposite of what a good thing to say to someone with cancer ought to do. However, the primary problem with most of those old cancer clichés is *they stop us from talking to each other about cancer.* Those long silences the cancer clichés facilitated was not the *mutual refraining from chatter* kind, the *respectful pause in conversation* kind, and not even the *I'll just wait now, because it's your turn to speak* kind. The silences were awkward, shocked, baffled and inappropriate. When we thought the person we said the things to was feeling comforted, they were more likely wondering if right at that moment it would be wholly inappropriate to poke us in the eye. Well, maybe not, but *just maybe* often enough for us all to be a little bit concerned about.

I'm not the authority on the things not to say to someone who has cancer, however, there is something I am an authority on. Every person with cancer, every person who ever had it, and every person who ever cared for a person who had cancer is an authority on this as well. It's *their story*. I am the expert on what happened to me, the way I felt about it and the way I dealt with it, as is every single person diagnosed with cancer and the folks who love them. Much of what I've written here is based on my own experiences and those of the people I've met, cared for, worked beside, helped, been helped by and shared with. Our expertise is varied - about as widely as the scope of our experiences. Our perspectives vary as well, and I fully realize many people who have been affected by cancer don't think the things I've brought up in this book are particularly problematic. A lot of people I've spoken to wonder why I bring it up, because for them, cancer clichés and the strange things people sometimes say and do around a person with cancer are simply not a big issue. Perhaps they ignored those inappropriate things when they were said, or didn't give them as much thought as I have. I do know some people have told me they didn't consider the things not to say offensive enough to warrant a book, a website, and quite a few indignant blog posts. But more than a few folks have laughed and cried telling me the things that were said and done when they had cancer, things they wish they'd had the confidence to say something about at the time, but didn't feel like they could. The number of emails, messages and hits on my blog from people searching "Things Not To Say To Someone Who Has Cancer" also tells me where cancer is concerned, an awful lot of people feel the old ways of speaking and acting simply aren't working for them, and they, like me, are actively seeking new ones.

When it comes down to it, my biggest problem with the things not to say is the waste of a wonderful opportunity. In that precious moment of interaction between one person in a very frightening situation having been diagnosed with cancer, and another person probably just as frightened, where each one could probably help the other, there's an opportunity for a real connection to occur. But too many times, what is brought to this moment is what we think we're supposed to say, or something we've heard said before. Sometimes we're afraid to say nothing, so we just say the first thing that springs to mind. Unfortunately, and quite inadvertently, this can turn out to be the verbal equivalent of a house brick. *Here, I brought you this. I can't use it, don't know what you're supposed to do with it, but just as long as you don't look at it too carefully, it might actually seem like I did a good thing here.* So, what might happen if we all stopped trying to be brave and clever, and just allowed one another to say how we really felt? What if we pushed past the first scary moments, refrained from filling the air with platitudes and meaningless conversation and just permitted those yawning silences to hang there? What if we all just made up our minds it was far more important to be honest than to be strong?

This is what I'd like to find out.

I suspect what would happen is we would all begin to really understand what it's actually like to have cancer in the real world, and what it's really like to be a person who loves someone who has cancer. For too long, we've looked to things like the media and to the past to show us and tell us what to do, and both have made a shocking job of it, in my opinion. The headlines and images of cancer and the people who have it we've been referencing it are largely based on stereotypes and metaphors no longer relevant, living as we are in a world where cancer is not uncommon, or necessarily fatal.

A friend of mine practices alternative therapies and has many clients with cancer. Recently she lamented to me that despite the wide prevalence of potentially fatal diseases such as diabetes and heart disease, both of which carry mortality rates comparable to those of cancer, her clients still seem to fear a cancer diagnosis more than just about anything. "They immediately imagine themselves becoming thin, bald and bedridden, and head home to write a will. But when told they have heart disease, they take their doctors prescription to the chemist, make up their minds to join an exercise class and plan not to let it get in the way of their enjoyment of life. This disparity affects their perception of the power the disease has over them, and can even affect their ability to manage their symptoms effectively." I think she's right. Our collective cancer imagination, based as it is on an outdated mythology of fear and brutal war metaphors, is skewed and inaccurate, and our programmed responses only further perpetuate these myths and misnomers. We need a new cancer imagination, one based on the reality of the huge advances in research, growing awareness of what causes cancer, and the real quality of life of people being diagnosed and treated for cancer.

Not only are we the expert on our own experience, we are also the author; however we don't always exercise this authority we possess to recreate our own life narrative. We can't always choose what happens to us, but we do have the opportunity to decide what those experiences and circumstances mean for us and how we might move beyond them. Without a sense that we are the pilot, the navigator and the charter of our own life experience, we won't look for new ways to deal with issues when we're afraid or uncertain. Instead, we'll look to others or else face backwards to the past, orientating ourselves by what's been said and done before. When our lives are touches by cancer, we may feel vulnerable and out of control, and without a new narrative, many of us simply revert to what we think is expected. Unfortunately, the way cancer is generally portrayed and the terrible things we hear about it means that for most of us our predominant default setting for cancer is "total disaster". We may kowtow to it and treat it like an elephant in the room, but a great deal of who and what we are and what we have to do won't be different simply because cancer is present. Bills will still have to be paid. Children will still need to be raised. Relationships will still need to be maintained, and special occasions celebrated. Apart from the physical aspects, there are and always will be places cancer cannot touch, as the famous poem celebrates.*** However invasive cancer may be physically, as the author of our own experience we always retain the power to decide how much it will affect us, how much it will take from us, and how much of us will be changed by it. Cancer is not always our foe, or a ruthless enemy to be resisted at all costs. I have sometimes heard it described as a teacher. With this perspective, any changes and challenges cancer brings might not always be considered intrusive or to be resisted. How much differently would we all react to cancer if our default setting were "learn", and not "fight"?

*** "What Cancer Cannot Do" - versions of the poem attributed to an anonymous author appear in various books and on the Internet.

You may disagree with everything I've written in this book. You might have thrown it across the room more than once by now, just as I have with almost every book I've ever read about cancer or about someone that had it. I've disliked cancer books wholesale as a genre so much and for so long it's taken me a very long time to write one myself. I'm not so smug as to think there aren't a few folks out there who will think both my book and I are full of crap. That's perfectly okay with me. I'm good with you throwing this book across the room. I'm also okay with you not agreeing with me about the things I've said. Far more than I want to convince you my thoughts and conclusions are the right ones, I want you to think about it for yourself. I also want you to talk about it, and I want you to get excited about it, maybe even excited enough to throw this book across the room. I want you to explore the possibility you may have some preconceptions about cancer of your own, preconceptions that could affect the way you behave when you're around someone who has it, or when you yourself may be diagnosed with it. If I want anything to happen because of this book, I want us to think about *what we think* about cancer, and work out whether these thoughts and beliefs are based on reality and fact, or on something else. If all this book manages to do is go some way towards demystifying cancer and treatment, to start some conversations about it and give everyone permission to talk about how they really feel, I'll feel I've succeeded, even if the conclusions people come to after those conversations are the exact opposite to my own.

Bound up in every single cancer cliché is a little bit of truth and a little bit of good, but both have nothing to do with the actual words. The cliché's themselves often make no sense at all, but the reason we've continued to use them is because we have always really been able to see what's going on behind them. *Behind every cancer cliché is a person who cares enough to want to say something.* So, what would happen if we kept that part intact, and somehow lost all the impotent and redundant words? When we say "What doesn't kill you makes you stronger", don't we really mean, "I'm incredibly afraid you'll die, so I know you must be absolutely terrified. Let's both of us hope together something better is coming"? Now there's something we can talk about. There's something I as a person with cancer want to believe. There's permission for me to be afraid and weak, and also reassurance you'll be there as we walk this journey together. The difference between the former and the latter thing to say is certainly courage and mindfulness, but also honesty, and I know that can seem like a big ask when you're afraid and feel out of your depth. But you know what? When it comes to the person you love who happens to have cancer, I don't think you're as far out of your depth as you might think. *I think you can do this.* It'll be confronting, and it'll be challenging, but it will also be absolutely worth it, because you and all you bring are exactly what are needed in this situation. Even with all your fear and awkwardness, you are not the problem. Cancer is the problem, and you, I, and everyone else involved are actually part of the solution.

So, let me take this opportunity to thank you for reading this book. I'd like to celebrate you as well for having the courage to confront this subject and for believing that you might be able to change things for the better. I know you can. I'd also like to know what you think. I'd like to know your story. I'd like to know your "things not to say", and how you dealt with them, whether it was with humor or a poke in the eye. Tell me - tell us - your story.

Please visit my website at www.johilder.com or email me at mail@johilder.com and share your experiences. Let's teach and learn from each other. Let's create a new kind of cancer conversation, and let's show people through our creativity, our images and our stories what cancer is and is not. Let's agree to tell the truth, our truth, about cancer, and our experience of it, instead of merely allowing others to depict and shape us according to old stereotypes and clichés. When cancer comes it often brings fear and uncertainty, threatens to take away our health and vitality and to separate us from everything we care about. *Let's not let it.* If we must fight cancer, let's make the battle against the unnecessary fears we've held on to, and against the breakdown in communication those fears can cause. Let's fight against the mindsets and the perspectives that dictate cancer is bigger and stronger than we are, and nothing good can ever come of it. Let's stop cancer from making us into the ones that pay, socially, physically and emotionally – and *let's make cancer pay*. Let's flip cancer into something that can no longer rob, steal and destroy, but which brings with it greater opportunities for caring, learning and understanding. Let's make cancer into something that causes us to become closer and more honest with one another, instead of discordant and disenfranchised. Let's not become, or make others into, cancer victims or cancer heroes any more, and let's not place expectations on one another to be anything other than who and what we really are. Let's make cancer into an opportunity to tell - and live - our authentic truth, rather than cancer just being another face we wear or another category we fall into. Cancer, with all its connotations of death and destruction, has a power over us it does not deserve, and we can take that power back. How do we do this? As I mentioned before, by not allowing cancer to take anything away from us in any more ways than is absolutely necessary.

So, my whiteboard is quite full now, and we're all talked out about cancer at last. It's been a great conversation, and it's time for this particular session on things not to say to someone who has cancer to end. And to celebrate, I'm not declaring a war on cancer. I'm declaring a picnic. I'm inviting all the folks I care about to come to a big cancer party, a party where everyone has something in common – cancer. Remember, one in two people will be directly affected by cancer in their lifetime, so it's probably going to be a huge party. I'm cheating though, because I already know what happens at parties like this. I've thrown them before. Everyone thinks we'll be sitting around talking about cancer, but that's never what actually happens. We always find out we have far more in common than cancer, and so cancer becomes a very boring thing to talk about after a while. Before too long everyone starts talking

173

about far more interesting things. The conversation at these cancer parties, if we let them, always leaves off cancer and heads other places - places nobody ever seems to mind them heading. The conversations stop sounding like this –

"They said. They think. They found. They decided. They gave me. They want to. They told me. They know what they're doing. They don't know what they're doing..."

And they start sounding like this.

"I love. I fear. I feel. I want. I know. I learned. I believe. I see. I dream."

"I hope."

Now there's a thing to say to someone who has cancer if ever I heard one. ☺

Glossary of commonly used terms

Alopecia	Hair loss from head and/or other parts of the body.
Ambulant	Able to walk around and not confined to bed.
Alternative treatment	Treatments or medications not officially approved by medical or government therapeutic goods regulation agencies. May be used to describe treatments offered as a substitute for or addition to approved medical treatments.
Anemia	Blood condition indicating a deficiency of red blood cells.
Autologous	Where the donor of blood/blood products and the recipient of those products are the same person. E.g.: autologous blood transfusion or stem cell transplant
Benign	A tumor which is not cancerous or

	malignant.
Biopsy - needle	The insertion of a fine, hollow needle into tissue for extracting and testing a sample of cells.
Biopsy – bone marrow	Procedure for extracting a sample of bone marrow with a needle usually under a local anesthetic for testing.
Blastoma	A cancer created by malignancies in precursor cells (cells in the bone marrow that are no longer capable of self-renewal).
Carcenogenic	A substance directly associated causally with the formation or development of cancer.
Carcinoma	Cancer arising from membranous tissue covering internal organs and other internal surfaces of the body, or epithelial cells.
Chemotherapy	The use of drugs and/or medications to treat cancer by targeting the growth of fast-growing cancer cells.
Complementary	Healing or therapeutic practices falling

medicine	outside, or used to complement, standard treatments or conventional medicine.
CT Scan	Computed tomography – diagnostic procedure where a number of x-rays are taken of the body to produce cross-sectional images of internal organs.
Cytotoxic	Chemical substances toxic to living cells.
Endocrine	Relating to glands that secrete hormones or other products into the blood. E.g.: pineal gland, pituitary gland, thyroid, thymus, pancreas, ovaries, testes, and adrenals.
Gallium Scan	A procedure to detect rapidly diving cancer cells by injecting radioactive gallium into the body and then scanning with a detection machine.
Haematology / Hemotology	To do with blood and blood-forming organs.
Hepatomegaly	Abnormal enlargement of the liver.
Hospice	A facility which provides

	accommodation and care for the sick or terminally ill.
Invasive	Involving the introducing of instruments or other objects into the body or body cavities, or else the intrusive spread of disease throughout organs or tissue of the body.
Leukaemia / Leukemia	A group of cancers of blood-forming tissues.
Lymphocytes	A type of white blood cell that helps to fight infection in the body.
Lymph Node	Small ball-like organs occurring in the armpit, groin, neck and other parts of the body. Healthy lymph nodes act as filters to remove foreign substances including cancer cells remove cell waste and help fight infections, but can become hard and swollen in the presence of disease.
Lymphoma	Cancer of the lymphatic cells of the immune system.
Markers,	Substances found in the body when cancer is present, and measured using

Tumor/Cancer	blood and urine testing to diagnose cancer, determine cancer type, and sometimes to identify if treatment is effective.
Malignancy	Uncontrolled proliferation of cells of the body, cells with the ability to spread, invade and destroy tissue.
Mammogram	Imaging procedure of the soft tissue of the breast.
Melanoma	A malignant tumor of melanocytes, the cells that produce pigment in the skin. Mainly associated with skin cancer, but can be found in other organs in the body.
Mesothelioma	A type of carcinoma of the mesothelium - the lining of the lungs or abdomen or heart, commonly associated with exposure to asbestos.
Metastases	The spread of cancer to other parts of the body.
Monoclonal antibody	A type of manufactured protein that can locate and cling to the surface of cancer cells, used in various

	medications to treat cancer.
Morbidity (statistics)	When discussed in terms of statistics, morbidity means the incidence of a disease, concerning the percentage of a population affected. It doesn't mean how many people die.
Mortality (statistics)	The risk of death based on factors such as age, health, gender, and lifestyle.
MRI	Magnetic resonance imaging, a diagnostic imaging procedure for looking at internal organs and structures of the body.
Myeloma	Cancer of the protein-producing plasma cells of the bone marrow.
Oncology	The field of medicine dealing with cancer and tumors.
Palliative	Treatment which alleviates pain or the effects of symptoms, but which does not cure the disease or underlying cause.
Pathogenesis	The chain of events leading to and development of disease.

Pathology	The science of the various causes and effects of disease.
Peri-menopause	Transitional phase when a woman passes from a normal reproductive state to menopause sometimes brought on by chemotherapy.
PET Scan	Positron emission tomography – a diagnostic tool used to find cancer in organs according to how fast they metabolize sugar. This is based on the premise that cancer cells metabolize sugar faster than non-cancerous cells.
PICC line	Peripherally inserted central catheter – a form of intravenous line inserted into a vein, suitable for giving medications over a long period of time. E.g.: chemotherapy.
Polyps	An abnormal growth of tissue produced from a mucous membrane.
Portacath	A small medical appliance installed beneath the skin, usually in the chest, with a catheter connected to a vein, for administering medications such as

	chemotherapy over a long period of time.
PSA Test	Prostate-specific antigen test given to measure the level of a protein produced by the prostate which increases if the prostate is cancerous.
Psycho-social	To do with psychological health and well-being related to surrounding environments and conditions. Often used in relation to supportive care and counseling for people who have been through cancer.
Radiotherapy	The use of ionizing radiation to treat cancer by exposing the patient to short bursts of radiation to diseases areas over a prescribed period of time.
Sarcoma	A usually cancer of connective tissue such as bone or muscle.
Shingles	A viral disease caused by the herpes zoster or Chicken Pox virus, characterized by intensely itchy and painful blisters occurring in a band or rash across the body. Can occur when

	the immune system is compromised such as during cancer treatment.
Splenomegaly	Abnormal enlargement of the spleen.
Staging	Assessment of the extent of cancer used in diagnosis, using a scale of numbers usually 1 − 4 and letters A and B. Staging methods differ depending on the cancer.
Stem Cell Harvest	Painless collection of stem cells from bone marrow or blood via a blood filtering process similar to dialysis.
Stem Cell Transplant	Procedure involving infusing stem cells into a cancer patient in order to enhance or restore normal blood cell production.
Tumour, Tumor	Abnormal growth of cells of the body.
Ultrasound	Otherwise known as sonography, diagnostic imaging method using high-frequency sound waves to see organs and tissue structures inside the body.